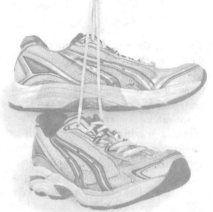

The "I Hate to " Exercise

Book for People with Diabetes

3RD EDITION

Charlotte Hayes, MMSc, MS, RD, CDE

American Diabetes Association.

Director, Book Publishing, Abe Ogden; *Managing Editor,* Greg Guthrie; *Acquisitions Editor,* Victor Van Beuren; *Editor,* Rebekah Renshaw; *Production Manager,* Melissa Sprott; *Composition,* ADA; *Cover Design,* Vis-à-Vis Creative Concepts; *Photographer,* Scavone Photography; *Printer,* Versa Press.

Printed in the United States of America
1 3 5 7 9 10 8 6 4 2

The suggestions and information contained in this publication are generally consistent with the *Clinical Practice Recommendations* and other policies of the American Diabetes Association, but they do not represent the policy or position of the Association or any of its boards or committees. Reasonable steps have been taken to ensure the accuracy of the information presented. However, the American Diabetes Association cannot ensure the safety or efficacy of any product or service described in this publication. Individuals are advised to consult a physician or other appropriate health care professional before undertaking any diet or exercise program or taking any medication referred to in this publication. Professionals must use and apply their own professional judgment, experience, and training and should not rely solely on the information contained in this publication before prescribing any diet, exercise, or medication. The American Diabetes Association—its officers, directors, employees, volunteers, and members—assumes no responsibility or liability for personal or other injury, loss, or damage that may result from the suggestions or information in this publication.

♾ The paper in this publication meets the requirements of the ANSI Standard Z39.48-1992 (permanence of paper).

ADA titles may be purchased for business or promotional use or for special sales. To purchase more than 50 copies of this book at a discount, or for custom editions of this book with your logo, contact the American Diabetes Association at the address below, at booksales@diabetes. org, or by calling 703-299-2046.

American Diabetes Association
1701 North Beauregard Street
Alexandria, Virginia 22311

DOI: 10.2337/9781580404938

Library of Congress Cataloging-in-Publication Data
Hayes, Charlotte, 1958-
  The "I hate to exercise" book for people with diabetes and pre-diabetes : turn everyday home activities into a low-impact fitness plan you'll love / Charlotte Hayes, MMSc, MS, RD, CDE. -- 3rd edition.
       pages cm
Includes bibliographical references and index.
ISBN 978-1-58040-493-8 (alk. paper)
1. Diabetes--Exercise therapy--Popular works. I. Title.
RC661.E94H34 2013
616.4'620642--dc23
                              2012038642

CONTENTS

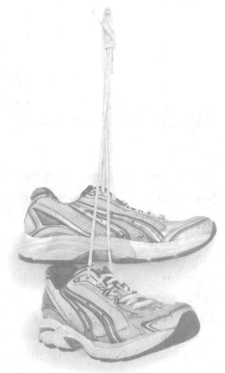

ACKNOWLEDGMENTS

Writing this book has been an endeavor that I could not have accomplished alone. Many people have coached me and cheered me along the way and have offered invaluable input.

I must first recognize my parents, who inspired my passion for promoting health. They have always placed high priority on healthy and vigorous living and have set excellent examples of how to age well. They have enjoyed cycling on the country roads of Wisconsin, nurturing a bountiful vegetable garden, giving tirelessly to their family, friends, and community—doing all this well into their 80s.

I have had exceptional mentors and colleagues throughout my career. Each of these individuals has graciously shared their knowledge, experience, and passion for making a difference to those living with diabetes. Thanks must go to my many friends and colleagues in the diabetes community who have offered encouragement, input, and expertise as I have written this book.

The dedicated and exceptional people in publications at the American Diabetes Association cannot go without recognition. Special thanks to Rebekah Renshaw, Victor Van Buren, and Greg Guthrie who have each offered guidance, support, and encouragement along the way. I cannot think of a more enjoyable group of people to work with throughout this project.

Finally, special thanks and appreciation must go to my husband and children for their support, encouragement, and patience, when I was hard at work writing and not wishing to be disturbed. They have been great sports and good comrades on the many evenings and weekends I dedicated to writing—often joining me to quietly read or study nearby. To Scott, JP, and Katie, I cannot imagine completing this work without your presence. Last but not least, to our Airdales, Beau and Aero, thank you for ensuring I accumulated a respectable number of steps each and every day. You are the best, most fun, "fitness buddies" I could ever have!

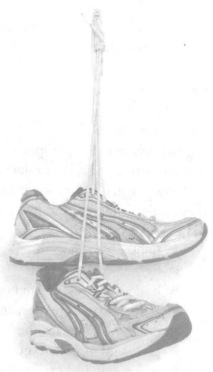

Chapter 1

WHY CARE ABOUT EXERCISE?

Good for you. Opening this book just burned a few calories. In fact, doing just about any activity burns calories. For instance, people who fidget burn more calories than people who just sit. So, wiggle your foot, tap your fingers, or rock in a rocking chair. When you're moving, you're burning calories.

Fidgeting isn't really exercise, and it won't bring you all the benefits that you want from real physical activity. But for most people, exercise is simply dreadful—something to avoid. Perhaps you hate exercise because you don't know how to do it. Perhaps the word exercise brings up a painful or embarrassing memory of junior high gym class. Perhaps you feel you're too overweight and out of shape to even imagine yourself getting up and doing anything. This book will show you that you're already doing things that can count as exercise—things you probably enjoy much more than gym class or fidgeting. And this book can tell you how to add activity to your day—while no one else will even know that you're exercising!

So what you're really asking is: how can I become a person who exercises and, more importantly, enjoys it? Read on.

Why Become More Active?

Exercise is the magic bullet, the perfect pill, and a solution to most health problems. People spend hours and many dollars shopping for lotions, potions, special products, and procedures to make themselves look good, when if they spent as little as 30 minutes a day being active, they could look good and feel great. Exercise is everything it's cracked up to be. Exercise

- boosts your mood;
- lightens your weight;
- builds muscles, which burn calories, even at rest;
- reduces stress, anxiety, and depression;
- improves your sex life;
- gives you more energy;
- makes you feel great;
- makes you look great;
- gives you a sense of accomplishment.

On the flip side, there are consequences to being inactive. There is a strong link between "sitting" your way through life and developing many of the chronic diseases we struggle with today, including:

- heart disease
- high blood pressure
- high blood fat levels
- obesity and overweight
- pre-diabetes
- type 2 diabetes

Chances are that if you already have pre-diabetes or type 2 diabetes, you also have one or more of these other conditions or you run a higher risk of developing them. No single pill can help prevent all of these, but exercise can. Like magic, you can transform your body, your health, and you. Exercise works on all these health problems equally well—and unlike most pills, it works without side effects.

But wait! There's more. Exercise supports healthy aging. In fact, with exercise, you can move gracefully through your years with the flexibility, agility, and strength to do all the things you need to do—and want to do. With exercise, you can be more fit and have a better quality of life all the way through.

Why are so many people inactive?

We don't have to move much anymore. Many of the chores and activities that used to fill people's daily lives with physical activity have been erased by modern technology. Elevators, dishwashers, washing machines, riding lawn mowers, remote controls, and computers—inventions like these have made our lives easier. Unfortunately, they've made our lives so easy that we must now take steps to increase our activity if we want to stay healthy. Our bodies are like machines—they must be used, and cared for, to stay in good working condition.

So what prevents us from keeping our bodies in good working condition? Simply put, many people say they don't exercise because they don't have the time, place, or exercising buddies to keep them motivated. Or they're afraid to start because they've never been good at it. Or, it's those memories of school gym class. No matter what their reasons may be, it seems the hectic pace of daily life is keeping people from being active.

Is there another way?

Yes. You don't have to change jobs or give up your free time to fit exercise into your schedule. You don't have to go to the gym or jog every day. In fact, you never have to do those things. The latest research has found that physical activity does not need to be vigorous or structured to be good for you. Everyday chores, work-related tasks, and leisure-time activities count, too. In 2008, the Physical Activity Guidelines for Americans were first published to offer guidance about types and amounts of activity that can greatly improve the health of all Americans—including you! These guidelines encourage Americans to do two things:

▶ Accumulate at least two and one-half hours [150 minutes] of moderate-intensity aerobic physical activity each week. Walking briskly, water aerobics, dancing, and bicycling are examples of moderate-intensity aerobic activities.

► Do muscle strengthening activities on two or more days each week. These types of exercises work the muscles in your legs, arms, shoulders, back, abdomen, and chest and make them stronger. Calisthenics, lifting weights, using resistance bands, and doing chores that require lifting, pulling, or pushing are examples of activities that strengthen groups of muscles.

When you have diabetes or pre-diabetes, doing at least two and one-half hours [150 minutes] of aerobic physical activity along with strengthening exercises two to three times each week can help improve your blood glucose control and heart health. Physical activity is key to reaching and maintaining a healthy weight. When it comes to losing weight and keeping unwanted pounds from creeping back on, doing more is better. If weight loss or maintenance is your goal, gradually work toward doing four to five hours [240 to 300 minutes] of weekly activity. No matter what, the trick to improving glucose control is to be active most days, leaving no more than two days in a row without doing some type of activity.

You don't have to go out and exercise for a long stretch of time. It is equally beneficial to do several short sessions of activity lasting for as few as 10 minutes each. If you are doing something that requires you to sit for a long period of time, for example working at your computer or watching an hour-long TV program, be sure to periodically get up and move around. Sitting for prolonged amounts of time has health risks! Breaking up lengthy periods of sitting with some casual movement has been shown to lower glucose levels as well as improve risk factors for cardiovascular disease.

You'll be surprised at how your minutes of activity can add up when you do short activity sessions throughout the day (along with making an effort to break up prolonged periods of sitting). The way you go about accumulating 150 minutes (or more) of activity over a week's time is completely up to you! For example, walking for 10 minutes three times one day plus doing 30 minutes of yard work the next day adds up to 60 minutes of activity. This is great progress toward a weekly goal of doing 150 minutes of activity. Activities that fit into your daily life—such as brisk walking, yard work, and gardening—are good for you, and can count toward your weekly total. Remember, sweating is not required.

If you haven't been very active up to this point, don't worry. It's never too late. In fact, people in their nineties who start lifting 1-pound weights put on muscle just like twenty-somethings do. There are a lot of health myths about what aging does to physical ability. Don't believe any of them. The truth is that staying active can help reduce limitations and improve overall health as you age. If you haven't been active, begin with just a few minutes of physical activity each day. Build up gradually by adding on a minute or two to your activity sessions every few days. Don't get impatient and push yourself too hard, or you may get too sore to enjoy yourself, or you might even injure yourself. Slow and steady wins the race. If you have been doing some activity, such as walking, but haven't been doing it consistently, commit to a regular routine. The amount of activity you do is more important than what you do. And doing something is always better than just sitting there and thinking about it.

What if you have pre-diabetes or diabetes?

Everyone can succeed at becoming fit and healthy, and having pre-diabetes or diabetes makes it even more important for you to be physically active. Exercise improves your body's ability to use insulin, which improves glucose management in many ways. Physical activity also helps relieve stress, lift depression, and brighten your mood. When you have a chronic disease, being active can make a huge difference. Exercise builds muscle, and muscle burns calories, even at rest. There is nothing better than exercise because it just keeps on improving your health!

Exercise your way to blood glucose management

If you have pre-diabetes or type 2 diabetes, regular activity improves your blood glucose levels. Exercise lowers blood glucose by taking glucose out of the blood to use for energy during and after exercise. It also helps lower blood glucose levels in other ways:

▶ Muscle cells become more sensitive to insulin, so they do a better job of storing and using glucose for energy.

- Liver cells become more sensitive to insulin, preventing the liver from producing too much glucose.
- Exercise increases the amount of muscle you have. Muscle uses glucose as an energy source even while you're at rest. More muscle means lower glucose!
- Exercise helps you lose weight and body fat and keep it off. No more yo-yo weight loss. If you are overweight, a loss of even 10–20 pounds can really improve blood glucose readings and overall health.

Exercise your way to a healthy heart

If you are inactive, you are at greater risk for developing cardiovascular disease. If you also have pre-diabetes or diabetes, your chances of developing heart disease, stroke, or other circulatory conditions are even higher. Regular physical activity works in several ways to keep your heart and blood vessels healthy.

- It strengthens your heart muscle. A strong heart does a better job of pumping blood throughout your body. This is especially important at times of stress when the demands on your heart are high.
- It lowers your resting heart rate. This reduces work for your heart.
- It lowers blood pressure. This also reduces work for your heart.
- It lowers total cholesterol levels, increases HDL (good) cholesterol, and lowers triglyceride levels in the blood. This reduces the risk that important arteries in your heart, or other areas of your body, will become blocked.

Exercise your way to weight control

Weight loss and maintenance is often an important goal for people with pre-diabetes and diabetes. Losing even a small amount of weight can improve your blood glucose levels. For people with pre-diabetes, losing weight and staying active can prevent or delay the onset of type 2 diabetes. For some people with type 2 diabetes, losing some extra weight, along with healthy eating and exercise, may mean they can stop taking insulin and other diabetes medications and control the disease with fewer medications. Too often, however, people try to lose weight just by cutting back on what they eat. They don't increase their activity at the same time. However, the pounds come off faster and stay off if you add exercise to meal planning. In fact, exercising when you're trying to lose weight

▶ helps promote fat loss and prevent muscle loss (you naturally lose muscle as you age, so exercise helps you hold on to it);

▶ boosts your metabolic rate (which means your body burns calories as heat instead of storing them as fat);

▶ helps you burn extra calories (for example, if you walk three miles in an hour, you may burn about 300 calories—or the calories in the sandwich you enjoyed for lunch—as opposed to the 60 calories you burn just sitting in a chair);

▶ helps reduce extra weight around your middle (which is especially important for reducing blood pressure, improving blood fat levels, and improving blood glucose levels);

▶ helps regulate your appetite;

▶ helps prevent lost pounds from creeping back on;

▶ helps reduce stress and anxiety that can lead to overeating (if you overeat as a way to cope with stress, you'll find that exercise is a better coping mechanism in many ways).

So, the good news is that when you add exercise to your life you can improve your blood glucose control and your overall health, as well as lose weight and keep pounds off. You don't even have to go to a fitness center or do vigorous exercise to get great results! You can get the same benefits just by fitting moderate activity into your daily routine.

What do you do first?

So, you want all the benefits being active can give you. Now what? While moderate activity, such as walking at a modest pace, is safe for most everyone, talk with your health care provider and diabetes educators about your desire to increase your level of activity. They can support you in this effort and help you come up with safe and enjoyable ways of increasing your activity level. Your provider might want you to have a thorough check-up before you begin exercising, especially if you have complications of diabetes or if you have been very inactive and plan to do an activity that is more vigorous than brisk walking. This is especially important if you:

- ▶ have coronary artery disease (CAD) or risk factors in addition to diabetes such as
  - ▶ high blood pressure
  - ▶ high blood fat levels
  - ▶ a family history of premature heart disease (in a male relative under 55 or a female relative under 65 years old)
- ▶ have peripheral vascular disease (poor circulation in your feet or legs)
- ▶ have had a stroke or are at risk for having a stroke
- ▶ have retinopathy (diabetic eye disease) or nephropathy (diabetic kidney disease)
- ▶ have peripheral neuropathy (nerve damage in the arms or legs— symptoms are tingling, pain, numbness or lack of feeling, and reduced sense of coordination or balance)
- ▶ have autonomic neuropathy (damage to nerves that help control body functions—symptoms include blood pressure drop when moving from sitting to standing, lack of sweating, and not being able to sense low blood glucose)

If you have complications of diabetes, some activities may be safer for you than others. Also, the way you do the activities may be modified so you can do them safely. This is especially true if you consider doing a high-intensity activity. Table 1-1 on page 9 lists activities that warrant caution if you have diabetes-related complications and gives some safe alternatives. Most moderate lifestyle activities—the type that the U.S. Physical Activity Guidelines encourage you to fit into your daily routine—are safe to do when you have complications of diabetes. So, don't consider your diabetes a barrier to becoming more active.

Looking at Your Outlook

Reading this book is a good sign that you are getting ready to take action. You are taking steps to understand the important role physical activity plays in your health and quality of life. Carefully consider the benefits of being physically active. Remember that exercise can help you

Table 1-1. Exercising Safely with Diabetes Complications

DIABETES COMPLICATION	CAUTION!	BENEFICIAL ACTIVITIES
Heart disease	Very strenuous activity Heavy lifting or straining, isometric exercises Exercise in extreme heat or cold	Moderate aerobic activity; activities such as walking, gardening, fishing Moderate dynamic lifting, stretching Activity in a moderate climate
High blood pressure	Very strenuous activity Heavy lifting or straining, especially with breath holding; isometric exercise	Most moderate activity such as walking, moderate lifting, weight lifting with light weights and high repetitions, stretching
Nephropathy (also refer to blood pressure guidelines)	Strenuous activities that raise blood pressure	Light to moderate daily activities such as walking, light household chores, gardening, water exercise
Peripheral Neuropathy	Weight-bearing activities, especially if high-impact, strenuous, or prolonged, such as walking a distance, treadmill exercise, step exercise, jumping/hopping, exercise in heat or cold, activities that require superior balance	Moderate activities that are low-impact (e.g., cycling, swimming, chair exercises, stretching), light to moderate daily activities, exercise in a moderate climate
Autonomic Neuropathy	Strenuous exercise, physical activity in hot or cold conditions; rapid changes in posture	Exercise in a supervised setting such as a cardiac rehabilitation program; light activity in a moderate climate
Retinopathy	Strenuous exercise, activities that require heavy lifting and straining, breath holding while lifting or pushing, isometric exercise, high-impact activities that cause jarring, head-low activities	Moderate activities that are low-impact (e.g., walking, cycling, water exercise), moderate daily chores that do not involve heavy lifting, straining, or the head to be lower than the waist
Peripheral vascular disease	High-impact activities	Moderate walking (may do intermittent exercise with periods of walking followed by periods of rest), non-weight-bearing exercise: swimming, cycling, chair exercises
Osteoporosis or arthritis	High-impact activities	Moderate daily activities, walking, water exercise, resistance exercise (e.g., light lifting activities), stretching

lose weight and keep off pounds, improve your blood glucose control, improve your heart health, and increase your feelings of well-being. You may have additional reasons of your own. For example, you may want to keep up with your children or grandchildren.

The Importance Scale

Consider the Importance Scale. Point to the number on the scale that describes how important physical activity is to you (with 0 being not at all important and 10 being very important).

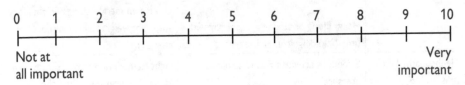

If you chose a number between 0 and 3...

You may not be convinced physical activity is as important as it really is. If this is true, keep reading about the many benefits of physical activity, as well as why leading an inactive lifestyle can have some serious consequences when it comes to your health.

If you chose a number between 4 and 6...

You probably consider physical activity somewhat important, but other things may be competing so it's not quite a priority. Consider making a list of reasons why becoming more active would be important to you. Then, make a list of reasons why becoming more active may not be a top priority. Consider what would change your thinking and make physical activity a greater priority.

If you chose a number between 7 and 10...

You are convinced that fitting exercise into your lifestyle is a priority for you. Now it's time for you to give it a try and start taking small steps to build a physical activity gameplan that will lead to success.

The Confidence Scale

A lot of people don't realize how important self-confidence is to exercise. People who have not been physically active often lack the confidence that they need to become more active, even if they know it is important for their health. The reasons for this lack of confidence are numerous and include health concerns; beliefs that exercise has to be painful to be beneficial; misconceptions that you have to wear tight-fitting clothes and go to a gym; or the notion that being physically active requires skill or takes a lot of time.

Consider the Confidence Scale below and point to the number on the scale that describes your level of self-confidence regarding doing physical activity (with 0 being not at all confident and 10 being very confident).

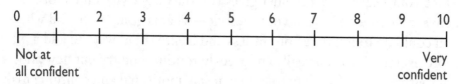

If you chose a number between 0 and 3...

You lack self-confidence, or certainty, that you have what it takes to become more physically active. You may feel that too many obstacles or roadblocks are in your way. If this is true, remember this bit of advice: Don't just look at the obstacle; look at the way around it.

Many times we look at reasons why we can't make lifestyle changes without ever looking for ways we can succeed. We become so focused on the obstacles that we don't ever look for ways around them.

So, list the reasons (or obstacles) that you think prevent you from becoming more physically active. But don't stop there! Next, list at least one way that you can overcome each obstacle. If you can't figure out a solution, read on for some tips on overcoming obstacles. Many of these techniques can help you achieve great success in your quest to become more physically active.

If you chose a number between 4 and 6...

You are fairly certain that you can become physically active, but you have some doubts. You may be concerned about a couple of obstacles that could get in your way. Remember: Don't just look at the obstacle; look at the way around it.

So, list the possible obstacles you feel are standing in your way, then figure out one or two strategies to help you work around them. Give one of these strategies a try. If it works, great! If not, adjust your strategy or try another one that results in success and boosts your confidence.

If you chose a number between 7 and 10...

You have a gameplan in place, and you're confident that you can fit exercise into your lifestyle. It's time for you to get started!

Looking at Your Lifestyle

Once your health care provider gives you the okay to become more active, take time to look at your lifestyle—what is going well, and what you could do to improve your fitness and health. Find ways to add a bit more exercise into your daily and weekly routine, and try out new and alternative types of activity to help you stay motivated and continue making progress toward becoming more fit. If doing things with others is something you enjoy, enlist the help of supportive people in your life.

How do you manage your time?

One of the great things about physical activity is that it can fit naturally into your day. Look at your daily routine to pinpoint times when you can realistically take a few minutes to do some activity. Ten minutes here or there can make a big difference. For example, you can:

▶ get up 10 minutes earlier than usual and do some stretches
▶ park a distance from your final destination and walk for an extra 10 minutes
▶ use the stairs instead of elevators or escalators
▶ take a 10-minute stroll after lunch or during a break from work
▶ spend 10 minutes doing some strengthening and stretching exercises before you retire for the night.

A little planning ahead allows you to slip activity into your day with ease. Of course, you need to be honest with yourself. If you are not a morning person, and dislike getting up early, don't schedule exercise time before you normally get out of bed. You will most likely sleep through your alarm or roll over and go back to sleep instead of getting up to exercise. Holidays, vacations, or demanding times with work or family can squeeze your time and make extra planning necessary. When you have to cut back, remind yourself that doing something, even if it's less than usual, is always better than doing nothing.

Tobacco use

You don't need a doctor to tell you that using tobacco is not healthy. Tobacco not only harms your health, but it can also make physical activity unpleasant and even painful. For example, if you smoke, you may have great difficulty climbing a flight of stairs, leaving you completely out of breath before you reach the top. The immediate discomfort you feel could keep you from taking the stairs the next time and send you right back to the elevator. If you can cut back on smoking—or better yet, kick your habit completely—you'll be surprised at how good you feel and how much easier and more enjoyable physical activity becomes.

Eating

Healthy eating patterns are essential to good health and definitely influence how we feel and how well we function. Athletes and avid exercisers often talk about how important nutrition is for achieving peak performance. Healthy food is premium fuel for your body. [See Box: What is Healthy Eating?]

Though most of us are not athletes, healthy eating is still necessary for fitness, well-being, and our best daily performance. Healthy eating is also a cornerstone of optimal diabetes management. If your eating habits have been iffy, you may experience high and low glucose levels and feel sluggish. Donuts won't get you as far as oatmeal. Healthy eating and physical activity are a powerful pair. Together, they can lead to improvements in blood glucose readings, blood fat levels, blood pressure, and weight. As your blood glucose control and overall health improve, you'll begin to feel more energized and ready to be more physically active.

What is Healthy Eating?

While eating habits are personal and unique to each one of us, these are a few things anyone can do to eat more healthfully:

▶ Balance calories by keeping portions in check. Too much of any food, even a healthy one, can supply extra calories and contribute to weight gain.

▶ Increase daily intake of fruits, vegetables, and whole grains.

▶ Choose fat-free dairy foods.

▶ Reduce sodium (salt) by choosing foods with lower sodium numbers.

▶ Reduce sugary foods and beverages.

▶ Build a healthier plate using Choose My Plate as a guide: http://www.choosemyplate.gov/food-groups/

Gaining support from others

You may want to enlist the support of others as you strive to live a more active lifestyle. Involving supportive people in your exercise plan can spread the benefits around. Your family members, friends, neighbors, and coworkers can all reap the health benefits of being active by joining you. Exercising with others can be motivating and a lot of fun. In fact, the fun and social aspects of doing physical activity along with others can be what helps you stick with your plan at times when you don't feel like exercising. Phone calls and friendly reminders from others, who count on you to be there too, can provide the extra nudge that is necessary for success.

If you know someone who is committed to living a physically active lifestyle and has established a consistent activity routine, ask them for guidance and support as you are becoming more active. A good role model can understand the challenges you face, provide feedback about the progress you have made, and offer helpful suggestions about how to succeed with your activity goals. Participating in the online community (DOC) is another way to gain support and share with others. The DOC is a place where you can connect with a virtual community of others with diabetes and learn and share as you strive to become more active and fit.

Even if the significant people in your life do not participate in the activity themselves, you need their support. Sometimes you'll need to ask others to adjust their schedules so that you can fit physical activity into yours. For example, if you plan to exercise early in the morning, you might ask your significant other to prepare breakfast. You may ask coworkers whether they can be flexible about their lunch schedules so that you can walk during your lunch break. Enlisting support before you set your activity goals is a good idea so that everyone can agree ahead of time on a plan that allows you to fit activity into your routine.

While exercising with others is usually helpful, don't feel like you can't also exercise alone. Depending on other people may not be what you want to do. If you had a busy day, you might need to find a different time to fit activity in. Or, some days, you may want some time alone to think and reflect on your day. These are two instances when exercising alone would be beneficial to you.

Today, many convenient health and fitness apps are available for download and use with your smartphone. These apps can help you keep track of your fitness routine and can also be very motivational. Plus, you don't have to depend on anyone else when you use them. It is really up to you to decide how and when to include other people in your fitness routine.

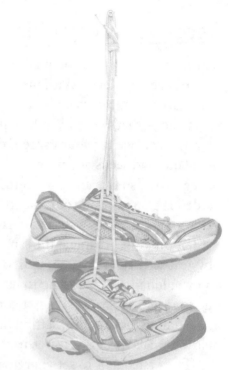

Chapter 2
GO FOR YOUR GOAL!

Just do it! You've probably heard that before, but it's the first step toward physical activity success. However, don't do it all at once. If you plan to hike five miles up a mountain for your first attempt at exercise, you'll probably come home discouraged. A more realistic way to start would be to walk a comfortable distance to the end of your block and back again, for example. By being kinder and gentler with realistic expectations of what you can accomplish, your first activity session will be much more enjoyable and successful. You'll feel energized by the activity rather than completely worn out, and you'll look forward to your next exercise session rather than just being relieved that the chore is over. Best of all, you'll experience a sense of satisfaction because you have done what you set out to do.

That feeling of accomplishment is very important when you are starting to increase activity. When you have reasonable expectations and set activity goals that you can achieve, success is sure to follow. Experiencing success is not only satisfying, it is very encouraging; it will help you establish a commitment to just do it—and to keep on doing it.

Setting Activity Goals

Setting goals can help you make gradual, steady progress toward increasing your activity level. With many things we do in life, we create a plan. Take gardening, for example. Let's say you want to grow your own fresh vegetables—that's your overall goal. Your plan would include deciding on a sunny place for your garden, tilling and preparing the soil, buying the plants and seeds you need, and deciding when to plant various types of vegetables so that the garden thrives from spring until fall. Once the garden is planted, you continue to do many carefully timed tasks, such as weeding, pruning, watering, fertilizing, and harvesting to keep the garden thriving. It's much the same when you set a goal for increasing physical activity. It's not enough to say, "I am going to exercise," just as you wouldn't say, "I'm going to have a vegetable garden" and then expect one to magically grow. When it comes to making lifestyle changes, such as becoming more active, setting SMART goals, or detailed plans, can help you make progress toward achieving healthier lifestyle habits.

The first step is to set your goal. Give it a try and see if you can achieve what you set out to do. If you find that you are successful, great! If not, then consider what went well and what did not work for you. Next, revise your SMART goal—trying out a new option that you think will work better. Keep trying until you figure out a plan that leads to success. By being detailed yet flexible, SMART goals can help you make progress with physical activity just as a well-made plan ensures a thriving and bountiful garden.

Let's take a look at how to set a SMART goal and then give it a try. Each letter in the acronym SMART has a specific meaning and purpose and is important to setting yourself up for success. So, this is what SMART means:

Specific—What exactly is it that you want to achieve? Clearly describe **what** you are going to do, **when** you will do it, **where** you will do it, and even with **whom**.

Measurable—How will you measure your progress and know that you have achieved your goal? Define **how much** you will do each time you exercise and **how many** days per week you will exercise.

Attainable—How certain are you that you can achieve your goal? A goal that is SMART is realistic—not perfectionistic. Though you will want to challenge yourself a bit, your goal should be set at a level you are pretty certain you can accomplish. Go back to the confidence scale on page xx. Your level of confidence should be a "7" or higher on the scale.

Relevant—How important is this goal to you? A goal should be something that matters to **you** (not just to somebody else), and it must be worth the effort it will take for you to achieve it. Think about the importance scale on page xx and make sure the level of importance you give your goal is at least a "7" on the scale.

Timelined—When do you want to have accomplished the goal? A SMART goal has a timeframe and a target date for completion; otherwise it is too easy to put it off. Aim for making weekly or even daily goals that will help you make step-wise progress with your physical activity routine.

Here is an example of a SMART goal:
"This week, I will walk three times for at least 20 minutes. On Monday and Wednesday I will walk outside during my lunch break, and on Saturday morning I will walk my dog at the park...."

Because this goal is specific (it outlines exactly when, where, and how much), measurable (it spells out how many times and for how many minutes), and timelined (it is a one-week goal), it will be clear if you are successful with accomplishing it or not. If for some reason you are not completely successful, you can evaluate barriers that have prevented you from completely achieving what you had set out to do. This also gives you an opportunity to consider alternatives and modify your goal so you will be more successful next time. By being flexible and willing to try alternatives, you are certain to develop goals that lead toward success with your exercise program.

One last thing: rewards are an important part of goal setting. Think of something special that you would like to reward yourself with as you reach goals and make progress with your physical activity plan. For example, watch a favorite movie, have a massage, save a dollar or two to put toward the purchase of new exercise clothing, or allow yourself time to do something you enjoy. For some, giving yourself a reward may seem uncomfortable; However, it can help you "keep your eyes on the prize" as you work toward your goal of becoming more active, fit, and healthy.

Setting an example: Jen

To illustrate how you can set SMART goals, let's visit Jen—and see how she used SMART goals to learn about herself and how to fit physical activity into her routine. Jen was recently diagnosed with type 2 diabetes. Like a lot of people, she did very little physical activity. At work she spent most of her time at her computer. In the evening, she prepared dinner and did some light household chores, then spent time online or watching TV. Jen realized that she would be healthier and feel better if she lost a few pounds and got her blood glucose and blood pressure into healthier ranges. She read some information online about the health benefits of doing moderate physical activity and decided she would like to build up to doing 30 minutes of activity most days of the week. Like many busy adults, Jen had trouble figuring out where to start and how to make progress toward her goal over the next few months. To overcome the first hurdle—getting started—Jen decided to make a detailed plan.

Jen's plan

Since she wasn't used to routinely exercising, Jen figured that doing 30 minutes of activity every day was probably too much to start with. Instead, she thought about what she could realistically do tomorrow. She felt quite sure that she could comfortably do two activity sessions, each lasting for 10 minutes. She knew that the activity should feel good and be energizing; it should not be so tiring and painful that the thought of exercise made her cringe.

Jen decided to take a "one day at a time" and "one week at a time" approach. She knew that by thinking short term she could build up, step-by-step, to doing 30 minutes of activity on most days. She also knew that by taking this approach she could achieve small victories along the way, which would encourage her to keep going.

Next, Jen developed SMART goals for the coming week:

1. I will walk for 10 minutes before lunch and 10 minutes in the evening on Monday, Wednesday, and Saturday this week.

2. On Monday morning, I will tell my coworkers that I am going to begin walking at lunchtime and will ask them to join me.
3. This weekend, I will talk with my family about my plan to do physical activity at home during the evenings and I will ask them to join me and work with me to become more physically active.

By setting her goal for three out of seven days, Jen knew she was creating a flexible plan and was avoiding "all or nothing" thinking. If she didn't manage to be active every day, she wouldn't feel like she was breaking away from her plan. Jen also knew it was important for her to gain support from others. She was uncertain how conversations about her physical activity plan would go with her family and coworkers. She knew it would be easy to not have these conversations. She also realized it was much more likely that she would talk to her colleagues and her family if she had specific SMART goals.

Next, Jen considered incentives. She enjoyed getting a manicure on Saturdays but had always considered this to be a bit of a luxury. As a reward for accomplishing her weekly activity goal, Jen decided to reward herself with a manicure when she achieved her goals.

Jen eventually worked up to doing 30 minutes of walking on most days. It took her several months to get to that level and, despite her best efforts, Jen didn't *always* achieve her weekly goals. A few times, her work schedule did not permit her to walk at lunchtime as planned, and at other times, her family's busy schedule created some barriers to her success. Jen learned to be flexible, to avoid feeling frustrated, and came up with a modified "plan B" at these times.

By setting weekly, achievable, SMART goals she stayed focused and positive, made gradual progress, enjoyed the activity that she did, and successfully accomplished what she had hoped to do. In addition, Jen's blood glucose and blood pressure levels improved, and she even lost some weight. Best of all, she felt healthier and more energetic—and enjoyed the satisfaction of her success!

Strategies for Success

Setting SMART goals and making a plan are first steps toward committing yourself to exercise. Staying committed is another thing altogether. If you have tried to maintain an exercise program before, you know how difficult it can be to "stick with it." What follows are some strategies for keeping yourself on track in achieving your fitness goals.

Make a contract

A good way to stay on track is to make your commitment more concrete. A physical activity contract is a written and signed agreement that states your activity goals and how you plan to accomplish them. The purpose of the contract is to help you stay committed to increasing physical activity and to remain focused while you work to reach your goals. It is an agreement that you make with yourself, so once you write the contract, sign it. You might ask a friend or another supportive person to sign it as well. The idea is that when you involve another person in your contract, you not only make a public statement about your activity goals, you ask the other person to help you uphold your agreement with yourself. (But remind the other person that nagging is not part of the job!) This adds weight to your contract, increases your sense of commitment, and enlists the help of individuals you can turn to if you have difficulty achieving your goals. A well-written contract:

▶ states your SMART goal(s);
▶ identifies how you will reward yourself;
▶ is signed and dated.

Figure 2-1 shows a sample physical activity contract.

Jen's Lifestyle Contract

Let's look at how Jen used the Lifestyle Contract to motivate herself:

1. Jen decided on a reasonable time frame for accomplishing her SMART goal(s): "This is a 1-week contract. I will begin working toward the goal stated in this contract on June 16, and I will evaluate my progress toward achieving this goal on June 23."
2. Jen then stated her specific physical activity SMART goals for the next week: "I will walk for 10 minutes before lunch and 10 minutes in the evening on Monday, Wednesday, and Saturday this week."
3. Jen noted her level of confidence.

Figure 2-1. Sample Lifestyle Goal and Activity Contract

Timeframe of Agreement:

This is a _____ week contract. I will begin working toward my goal on _____ and will evaluate my progress toward achieving these goals on _____. I will remain flexible and willing to revise my goal(s) until I find a plan that gets results and leads to my success.

My SMART Goal:

Remember to include what activity you will do, when you will do it, where you will do it, and how much (e.g., number of steps or repetitions of an exercise or how much time you will accrue).

This week I will:

WHAT _____

WHEN _____

WHERE _____

HOW MANY _____

My Level of Confidence is: _____ (on a scale of 0 to 10 with 0 being not at all confident, 5 being somewhat confident, and 10 being completely confident)

Success Tracker:

	Level of Success	Comments
Monday		
Tuesday		
Wednesday		
Thursday		
Friday		
Saturday		
Sunday		

Success Scale: 0–5 scale with 0 being not at all successful, 3 being 50% successful and 5 being 100% successful

My Reward for Achieving My Goal(s):

_____

_____

Signed:

_____   _____
Your Signature   Date

_____   _____
Supportive Other Signature   Date

4. Jen wrote down how she would reward herself when she achieved her goal: "I will have a manicure on Saturday afternoon if I achieve my activity goal."
5. Jen gained the support of her husband and a friend at work. She signed and dated the contract and asked each of them to sign it to show their support.

With her signed physical activity contract in hand, Jen was a step closer to her fitness goals.

Keeping self-talk positive

Self-talk is the inner conversation that we all have with ourselves. This conversation is not only a reflection of our thoughts and emotions; it also has a strong influence on how successful we are at making lifestyle changes. Self-talk that is positive and upbeat leads to success; self-talk that is negative and distorted can get in your way. That's why it's so important to be aware of the conversations you have with yourself about physical activity. If you tell yourself, "I've never been able to stick with exercise. I guess I'm just too lazy to be in good shape," you are being too hard on yourself. This kind of inner conversation can prevent you from being successful.

Sometimes, it is helpful to consider where such negative thoughts come from. Maybe you were the kind of person who never had success with sports or the kind of person who did everything you could to stay out of gym class. Perhaps this formed your thinking about your ability to be physically active as an adult. Fortunately, you can turn negative self-talk into a positive and reinforcing conversation. A healthy, self-supporting statement might be, "I know that I'm no marathon runner and that's fine. Gardening and walking are activities I enjoy, and I can improve my health by doing them." Table 2-1 lists some discouraging thoughts that may seem familiar and offers examples of how to turn those negative conversations into positive pep talks. If you catch yourself having a negative internal conversation about exercise, remember that you have the ability to turn things around. Talk back to yourself with a positive response.

Table 2-1. Negative Thoughts and Positive Alternatives

Types of Negative Thought	Examples	Positive Alternative
All or nothing thinking	I didn't walk every day last week. I'm an exercise failure.	I walked 4 out of 7 days last week; made progress toward my goal.
Disqualifying the positive	The only reason I parked far away from the entrance to the store was because I couldn't find a close parking spot.	I'm glad I decided to park at the end of the parking lot because I was able to do some extra walking on the way into the store.
Over-generalization	I can't run, so I can't get enough exercise to do me any good.	I like to walk; it is a good, healthy activity for me to do.
Negative interpretation	My doctor wants me to have a foot evaluation before I start doing more activity. That must mean exercise is bad for my feet.	Because I have diabetes, I always have to take good care of my feet. I'm glad that my doctor is making sure that the activity I do is right for me.
Personalization	The weatherman has something against me. I was planning to walk, but it has been raining cats and dogs all day long. I just can't win.	You can never really predict the weather, so I'm glad I have a plan for doing exercise indoors on rainy days like today.

Is the effort worth the result?

Very seldom are things in life absolutely free. Even if you are fortunate enough to win the lottery, first you had to buy a ticket. When some people weigh the low cost of the ticket against the possibility of winning big, they decide the investment is worth the risk. Others figure that the chances of winning are so slim that the cost of a ticket is just money down the drain.

Every day, we make many similar cost/benefit decisions, especially when we think about making lifestyle changes. If we see the cost as being reasonable and the benefit—or what we'll get in return—as being worth it, we tend to move forward with making changes. But if the cost seems too high and the benefits are uncertain, we aren't as likely to make the effort. For this reason, doing a cost/benefit analysis—listing the pros and cons of making changes to see if you think the result is worth the effort—can be a helpful exercise.

Table 2-2. Sample Physical Activity Cost/Benefit Balance Sheet

COST	STRATEGIES TO DECREASE	BENEFIT	STRATEGIES TO INCREASE
Time	Do small amounts of activity at convenient times	Better health	Do regular activity
Discomfort	Keep activity light/moderate and comfortable	Feel better	Be moderate and consistent
Boredom	Do a variety of activities to gain fitness	More energy	Gradually increase activity
Inconvenience	Fit activity into work and home routine	Greater ability to do things I enjoy	Gradually "build up" to get stronger
Embarrassment	Do only what I know I can successfully do	Look better	Increase activity enough to lose weight and gain muscle
Unpleasantness	Be open-minded and try different activities to find some I like	Enjoyment	Do activity with friends; do outside activities on nice days
Expense	Do activities at home that don't require special equipment	Time with friends	Arrange to do activity with friends
Place to exercise	Find ways to do activity at work or at home	Manage stress	Plan activity "stress breaks" of stretching or walking
		Like the challenge	Set goals that are challenging but within reach

A sample cost/benefit analysis appears in Table 2-2. To start your own analysis, first list things that you consider to be the costs—or cons—about doing more activity. Some examples:

▶ Extra time it will take
▶ Need to change your routine
▶ Sore muscles or other discomfort you might experience
▶ Notion that you just don't like doing the activity

Then list all the benefits—or pros—of making the change, the things that you will gain from being more active. Some potential benefits:

▶ Feeling better
▶ Looking better
▶ Improved health and diabetes control
▶ Increased energy level
▶ Better mood
▶ Ability to do more of the things you want to do

Now, weigh the pros and cons, and think of ways to reduce the costs and increase the benefits. For example, you can help avoid muscle soreness by starting with light or moderate activity and gradually working up toward more vigorous activity. And you can make time for exercise by setting your alarm clock a little earlier each day or doing some activity during your lunch hour. Ultimately, your aim is to have a balance sheet that is long on benefits and short on costs.

Giving yourself cues

Cues are signals that trigger us to take action. An actor, for example, depends on cues to tell him the correct time to come on stage. A traffic light that turns red is a cue that tells us to stop the car. Advertisers target TV viewers with numerous cues in commercials. If you find your mouth watering in response to an ad for a piping-hot pizza, you are responding to a powerful food cue. This cue may send you straight to the refrigerator or to the phone to call for carry out.

Cues can be positive and helpful or they can be negative and obstructive (if you are trying to lose weight, for example, the pizza commercial could be bad news when it comes to healthy eating and weight management goals). They can definitely influence your success with doing physical activity. For example, if you plan to walk after work, putting your walking shoes just inside the front door can serve as a positive cue—when you see them, it's your reminder to walk. On the other hand, if the first thing you see when you get home is a comfortable chair and a TV remote, this can be a negative cue. You may find yourself plopping down in front of the television instead of going for a pleasant walk.

As you probably already know, negative cues can be pretty hard to overcome. The idea, then, is to create positive cues that remind you to do more activity throughout the day. Some positive cues:

▶ placing exercise clothing or walking shoes where you can see them
▶ having a friend or significant other call just before your activity time
▶ writing yourself notes as reminders
▶ hanging the dog's leash on the doorknob

At the same time, remove as many negative cues as possible. If you're a TV addict, hide the remote or unplug the set. If you usually go online when you get home, keep your computer turned off until after you have accomplished your daily activity goal.

Plan for the unexpected

Life is full of surprises. Even when you have every intention of meeting your activity goals, challenges can arise, and sometimes breaks in an activity routine are unavoidable. Vacation or business travel, times when your work or your family demands more of your time, periods of bad weather, and an illness or injury are challenges that face most of us from time to time. When you come to these bumps in the road, the decision to take a positive approach is vital to your success.

One helpful way to avoid getting off track is to plan ahead. Before challenging situations occur, create an alternative plan. You may have to be flexible about the time of day you do your activity, for example. Or you may have to re-evaluate your activity goals and set them at a more achievable level for a while. Even if you do less than your usual amount of activity, remember that doing something is always better than doing nothing. And be sure to keep your self-talk positive during challenging times. Avoid all-or-nothing thinking and feelings of failure. Sometimes it's necessary to remind yourself, "I'm doing the best I can."

Self-monitoring and keeping track

As part of your diabetes or pre-diabetes management plan, you're probably already keeping track of your blood glucose, the foods you eat, and how much and what types of medications you take (and if not, consider keeping track!). You may also be keeping track of your weight, especially if weight loss and maintenance are goals. Though keeping track takes some time and commitment, it has many advantages, one of the greatest being that it keeps you in touch with your own diabetes care. People who are committed to keeping track and monitoring their own progress tend to have the greatest success making and sticking with lifestyle changes long term. In other words, the benefits of keeping track far outweigh the costs. Adding an activity log to your records also has benefits, since the information you collect can help you make decisions about how to achieve your physical activity goals. An activity log can

- ▶ measure your daily successes and challenges;
- ▶ track your progress toward achieving long-term activity goals;
- ▶ increase your awareness of your activity-related thoughts and feelings;

- increase your feelings of satisfaction and enjoyment related to doing activity;
- prevent relapse by helping to identify sticking points and early signs of a drop-off in activity;
- aid with troubleshooting by helping to identify alternative or better ways of fitting activity into your lifestyle.

Figure 2-2 shows a sample form for keeping track of activity. Since keeping a record should also be fun and easy, feel free to modify the form

Figure 2-2. Sample Activity Record

	Sun.	Mon.	Tues.	Wed.	Thurs.	Fri.	Sat.
ACTIVITY							
Type							
Time							
# minutes total							
RPE*							
ENJOYMENT							
1. Very +							
2. Somewhat +							
3. Neutral							
4. Somewhat −							
5. Very −							
SUCCESSES/CHALLENGES							
Self-Monitoring							
Blood glucose:							
Heart rate:							
Blood pressure:							
ACTIVITY GOAL ACHIEVED: Y/N							

*RPE = Borg Rating of Perceived Exertion Scale (See Figure 3-1)
+ = positive − = negative

King, A.C., and J.E. Martin. *Resource Manual for Guidelines for Exercise Testing and Prescription.* Dustine, J.L., et al., Eds. The American College of Sports Medicine, 2nd ed, Philadelphia; Lea and Febiger, 1993: 443–454.

Chambliss HO, and King AC, Behavioral Strategies to Enhance Physical Activity Participation in *ACSM's Resource Manual for Guidelines for Exercise Testing and Prescription.* Ehrman JK ed. The American College of Sports Medicine, 6th ed. Philadelphia; Lippincott Williams & Wilkins, 2010: 696–708.

to suit your needs. As long as the log provides feedback about your progress and helps you create a lasting activity habit, it can be as simple or as detailed as you want.

Are you ready to go?

Changing your lifestyle is rarely easy, but using strategies such as setting SMART goals, making a contract, practicing positive self-talk, and using an activity log to help you keep track will help you get there. You may find that some of these strategies work for you while others don't. Just remember to stay positive and keep an open mind.

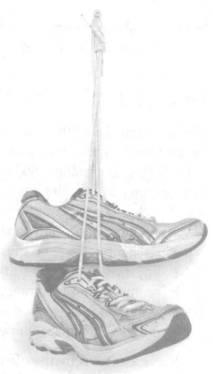

Chapter 3
BUILDING AN ACTIVITY PROGRAM

Be physically *in*efficient! That may sound strange, but it's the key to easily fitting in at least 30 minutes of activity each day. Simply identify opportunities to do things in a physically active—but not necessarily quick or easy—way. For example, give up the TV remote control so that you have to get up and move to change channels or to turn the TV on or off. By being more physically inefficient you can fit more activity into your daily routine, no matter how busy you are. By adding more minutes of moderate activity into most days to reach a total of at least 150 minutes of weekly activity, you can burn an extra 1,000 calories per week—a level of calorie burning that has health benefits. Increasing your amount of daily and weekly activity even more—by as much as 250 to 300 minutes per week—can help you to not only lose weight but more importantly to *keep it off*. However, don't worry about reaching this amount of activity right away. If you have not been doing any activity at all, simply start by doing something, no matter how little, and gradually build up from there. As your body and mind adapt to an active lifestyle, you will be surprised at the amount of physical activity you are able to do!

Get Your Muscles Moving

The large muscles of the body include the legs, arms, shoulders, and back muscles. When you do activities such as walking, mowing the lawn, swimming, stair climbing, biking, or vacuuming, you use large muscles in a repetitive and continuous way. These types of activities can improve your health in a number of ways. They

▶ strengthen the individual muscles;
▶ strengthen the heart muscle;
▶ improve the body's ability to use oxygen efficiently;
▶ promote calorie burning, weight loss, and loss of body fat;
▶ help reduce blood glucose levels;
▶ improve stamina, endurance, and energy level.

Because these activities offer many important benefits, finding ways to do a few short sessions each day can be a good way to increase your level of activity. A few ideas:

▶ Walk more whenever possible
▶ Park your car farther away when shopping or at work
▶ Instead of putting your dog out in the yard, take him for a walk
▶ If you use public transportation, get off a stop or two early and walk the added distance
▶ Take your children or grandchildren out for a walk
▶ Challenge yourself with electronic fitness games, like Wii Fit™
▶ Schedule short walking breaks each hour and walk around your office or home for a few minutes
▶ If a destination is within walking distance, put away the car keys and walk instead
▶ Walk or march in place while watching TV or talking on the phone
▶ Give up remote controls and other energy-saving devices that prevent you from getting up and walking even a short distance
▶ Take a walk just for the fun of it

- ► Take the stairs instead of the elevator or escalator for at least one floor.
- ► Do your own yard work
- ► Do your own housekeeping
- ► If you have a stationary bicycle, ride it while you read or watch TV
- ► Choose hobbies like golf, gardening, swimming, walking, tennis, and dancing instead of watching TV, going to the movies, or sitting at the computer

Do enough, not too much!

Physical activity should feel energizing, not painful or overly difficult. There are a couple of ways to tell if you are doing enough activity without pushing yourself too hard. The simplest way is to do the "talk test." You should always be able to talk to someone while you are doing an activity. If you become so short of breath that you can't talk, that's a sign that you should slow down. Why? First, if the activity feels uncomfortable or difficult, you are less likely to stick with it. Second, if you do too much too fast, you may become fatigued or injured. So remember, be kind and gentle with yourself—especially when you are just beginning to increase activity in your daily routine. As you become more fit, you'll be able to do more exercise at a more vigorous pace.

Another way of deciding if you are exercising at a comfortable level is to rely on your own perception of how the activity feels. A scale called the Borg Rating of Perceived Exertion (RPE) Scale (see Figure 3.1) was developed as a simple method of rating how much effort you feel an activity requires while you are doing it. Many factors can influence your perception of how an activity feels, including your level of fitness, how rested you are when you begin the activity, and environmental factors like heat and humidity. The RPE scale reflects all these factors. The ratings listed on the scale are related to how hard your heart is working and how well your body uses oxygen during exercise.

Using this scale can help you do an activity at an enjoyable level without working yourself to the point that you'll never want to exercise again. When you do an activity, you shouldn't expect to feel 6 or 7 on the scale, or "very, very light." You want to feel a bit more challenged than that. On the other hand, the activity should not feel in the range of 17 to 20—"very hard" or "very, very hard"—either. That is too much effort and will probably be very uncomfortable. If the activity feels in the range of 12–14 on the Borg scale, or "somewhat hard," you are gaining health and fitness benefits from the activity without pushing yourself too hard.

Figure 3-1. Borg Rating of Perceived Exertion (RPE) Scale

Least Effort

6	
7	Very, very light
8	
9	Very light
10	
11	Fairly light
12	
13	Somewhat hard
14	
15	Hard
16	
17	Very hard
18	
19	Very, very hard
20	

Maximal Effort

Borg, G.A.. Physiologic basis of physical exertion. *Med Sci Sports Exerc* 1982; 14: 377–387.

All of your body's muscles, even small ones, benefit from being called upon to do some work. Resistance exercises that require your muscles to push, pull, or lift can help strengthen specific muscles or groups of muscles. Make it a point to include these activities in your physical activity routine. Examples of resistance activities include light weight lifting, moderate calisthenics, and strengthening exercises that use resistance bands. These activities

▶ increase muscle strength;
▶ improve muscle tone;
▶ help reduce risk of osteoporosis and bone fractures;
▶ help improve balance and reduce risk of falls;
▶ increase muscle mass and help with weight control;
▶ increase energy level and improve fitness;
▶ increase the body's sensitivity to insulin.

You don't have to purchase special equipment to do these activities unless you wish. In fact, you probably have a set of weights already! You can use items like water bottles or cans of food as weights. Just lifting the weight of an arm or leg against the pull of gravity can work your muscles, so you may not even need any extra resistance at first. Later, as you gain strength, you can experiment with simple "equipment" to make resistance exercise more challenging. You can do many strengthening activities even while sitting in a chair (page 110), so try them while you watch TV, talk on the phone, or take a break at your desk during the workday.

In going about many of our routine daily tasks, most of us already do some resistance activities, for example:

Lifting

▶ Carrying a briefcase or purse
▶ Bringing a load of groceries into your house
▶ Taking the day's trash outside

Pushing

▶ Mowing the lawn
▶ Pushing a child in a stroller

Pulling

▶ Weeding your garden
▶ Pulling a child in a wagon
▶ Towing a cart or suitcase

In addition to helping you complete your daily chores, all of these activities help keep muscles strong. So don't shy away from doing them!

Of course, how you do resistance exercise is very important. Doing too many of these activities, doing them in the wrong way, or working against too much weight can lead to injury—and with injured muscles, it's hard to make progress with your exercise routine! To perform resistance activities safely:

▶ Keep it comfortable
▶ Start slowly and gradually build up
▶ Do slow, steady, controlled movements
▶ Avoid jerking or straining

- Correctly position your body for the exercise
- Focus on breathing (avoid holding your breath!)
- Cut back if you feel pain, soreness, or stiffness

Stretch and Relax

Stretching is very simple and easy to do. It requires little preplanning, and doesn't require special equipment. In fact, some forms of activity, like yoga, focus on stretching. Stretching is something that you can do nearly any time and almost anywhere. So, take a few mini-breaks throughout the day to do a few stretches and you will find you feel less tense and more relaxed. You will soon look forward to opportunities to stretch!

As an important part of a well-balanced activity routine, stretching provides a number of important benefits:
- increased flexibility
- increased range of motion of joints
- reduced stiffness

Stretching Do's & Don'ts

Like any exercise, there is a right way and a wrong way to stretch. Stretching should feel mild and relaxing, not uncomfortable and painful.

Do:
- Relax as you stretch
- Stretch only to the point that you feel mild tension
- Hold a steady stretch for 10–30 seconds
- Breathe deeply and slowly
- Keep it comfortable
- Ease off the stretch if you feel discomfort

DON'T:
- Bounce or bob
- Focus on tension-creating thoughts
- Hold your breath
- Strain or push to the point of pain

- reduced risk of muscle and joint injury
- reduced risk of developing back pain
- relief of muscular pain and tension

Build Balance and Agility

Balance is the ability to maintain body position when you stand or move about. Having good balance (when standing or walking) can keep you from stumbling or falling and injuring yourself. Agility is the ability to do activities with a spry quickness, and that's a big plus!

All types of activities—including walking or other large muscle movements, strengthening, and stretching activities—can help improve balance and agility. However, special exercises that are intended to improve balance can help even more. There are two types of balance activities—those that you do while standing still and those that you do while walking or moving.

Standing balance activities

1. Stand for a minute or so with your feet about 2 feet apart. If this is hard to do at first, support yourself with one hand on a countertop. Keep practicing until you are able to stand with steadiness and good balance without support.
2. As your balance gradually improves, move your feet closer together. Your goal is to stay steady and balanced when standing with your feet together.
3. Once you reach this goal, practice balancing on one leg and then the other. Again, support yourself with one hand on a countertop until you are able to balance on one foot without support.

Walking balance activities

1. Practice your normal walking pattern until you feel very stable.
2. Next, practice taking a few steps on an imaginary straight line by placing one foot directly in front of the other. Gradually increase the number of steps you are able to take.
3. When you have good balance doing this, practice taking heel-to-toe steps on the imaginary line.

How Long Should Each Activity Session Last?

It's up to you to decide how long an activity session lasts. Of course, many factors can influence the amount of time you spend exercising, such as time limitations, your level of fitness and conditioning, and how difficult an activity is for you to do. For example, you may be able to walk comfortably for 20 minutes and have time to do this during your lunch break. However, if you decide to climb the stairs to your office in the morning you may find that one flight is the most you can do at first. Or you may be rushed for time in the morning and decide to squeeze activity into a shorter session for this reason. As you gain fitness and skill at fitting activity in, you may decide to increase the length of either session.

Remember to look for opportunities to do things in an active way throughout the day. You can, at any time, benefit from moving more and doing brief sessions of stretching or light calisthenics—even without getting up out of your chair. Short sessions add up, and each one contributes to a daily activity total.

Be Active All Day!

Squeeze as much activity into a day as you comfortably can. Remember, the ultimate goal for improved health is to build up to doing at least 150 minutes (2 1/2 hours) of activity over a week's time and to go no more than two days in a row without doing any type of exercise. Remember to also "break up" sitting for long amounts of time. Get up and move around every so often to do a few stretches or strengthening exercises, or a few minutes of walking. Find ways to do things in a more energy inefficient way throughout the day.

Here is an example. On weekends, you may enjoy walking with a friend and decide to walk together for 30 minutes and then do some stretching afterward. In this case, you are able to make good progress toward your weekly activity goal in just one session. During the week, you may choose to do shorter sessions of activity. For example, if you walk your dog for 10 minutes in the morning, take a 10-minute walk during lunch, and do 15 minutes of stretching and strengthening activities in the evening, you've accomplished 35 minutes of activity. Just how you accumulate activity time throughout the week is up to you. You can either do short (10-minute) sessions frequently or longer sessions less frequently. The most important thing is to be creative and flexible in finding ways to achieve your activity goals.

Building on Your Exercise Foundation

Now you have the material that you need to start building a daily activity routine that you find to be not just realistic but also energizing and enjoyable. Remember, there are three types of activities that are the foundation of any well-planned daily routine:

▶ Large muscle movement activities (such as walking)
▶ Resistance or pulling, pushing, and lifting activities (such as using resistance bands, weight lifting, or doing exercises like sit-ups or push-ups)
▶ Stretching activities

Your first task is to look at each day and figure out how to best fit in an activity at any given time. For example, if you have the option of walking down the street to visit a neighbor or driving your car, take the active option. Use your large muscles and walk. If you have the choice of pushing your own cart out of the grocery store and loading your groceries into your car or of having someone do it for you, take the active option and do the pushing and lifting yourself. It is a great opportunity to keep muscles strong without taking up a lot of time. When you watch TV at night, you can either sit passively or you can do some stretching or strengthening while you watch. Build some activity in. It will feel great and it doesn't cost any additional free time.

Each of these types of activities can fit into your routine in a unique way, just as each type offers its own special set of benefits. The following chapter presents specific ideas on how you can fit physical activity into each day. Draw upon these ideas, experiment, and try them out so that you can become physically active in your own way.

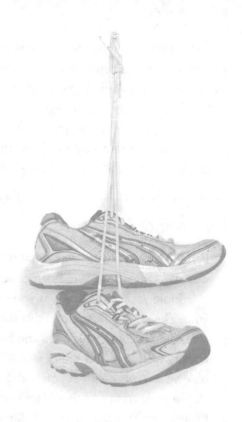

Chapter 4

BE ACTIVE EVERYWHERE

Most of our daily life is spent in three places: at home, at work, and out and about in the community. Fortunately, all three settings offer a variety of opportunities to be physically active. At home, you can work light exercise into household chores, yard work, and family time. At the office, a short activity break can be a welcome relief from the day's stress. Out in the community, you can mix exercise into running errands or going out for entertainment. A little bit of planning, including some daily activity in these three areas of your life, can result in benefits that add up to boost your level of fitness. You are limited only by your imagination.

Getting the Most Out of Everything You Do

You can reap physical gains from doing even the simplest task. The trick is to focus on doing it in an active and vigorous way. For example, when you mow the lawn or vacuum the floor, pick up the pace a little bit to give your heart a better workout. Actively push and pull with your arms and shoulders so that they benefit and get stronger from the work. When you unload the clothes dryer or prepare to hang laundry out on the line, bend your knees a little more than usual as you pick up the items. This will help strengthen your leg muscles. And as you hang clothes on the clothesline, reach and stretch a little farther than usual. This will help increase upper body strength and flexibility. Almost any task can be beneficial if you go about it in an active and vigorous manner.

Active and Vigorous?

If you're not quite clear on what doing things in a more "active and vigorous" way means, here is a demonstration you can try:

Hold your arms down at your sides so that they are relaxed and limp. Then, keeping them in this fairly floppy state, lift them out to the side, then up over your head and back down to your sides. How did the activity feel? Probably didn't feel like much work for your muscles. Now, hold your arms down at your sides again, only this time tense the muscles in your arms and shoulders and point your fingers down to the floor. Maintaining this tension, slowly lift your arms up. (Think about stretching and reaching for the walls as you lift your arms to the side, then overhead toward the ceiling.) Take a deep breath in as you reach up. Then, while maintaining this tension and energy, return your arms to the starting position, breathing out as you do this. How did the activity feel this time? Did you feel your muscles working? Did you feel a good stretch? Did you feel invigorated as you breathed in deeply and then exhaled? The answer is probably, "Yes!" That is the benefit of doing even routine tasks in an active and vigorous way.

Being Active at Home

There is no place like home, especially if you're looking to become more physically active. Your home offers the most options for fitting activity into your day. Each work-related task or leisure activity you do has the potential to benefit you in a variety of ways. For example, if you enjoy cooking and baking you can give your arms, shoulders, and back a workout—especially if you vigorously move as you go about tasks such as chopping, stirring, kneading, pushing dishes into the oven, or pulling them back out and lifting pans off the stove. If you take your dog for a walk in the evening, you will gain very different benefits: Walking uses large muscles in your legs and exercises your heart muscle as well. But unlike cooking and baking, walking doesn't give your upper body much work to do. So walking and working in your kitchen each offer unique benefits in terms of which muscles they use and how they use them. A key point to remember is that if you do both activities in a day, you get all the benefits! This is why doing a variety of tasks that require you to use your muscles, both at work and at play, is so desirable.

The number of calories burned is significantly different between walking and cooking or baking. Table 4-1 looks at chores that most of us do at home and the average number of calories burned in 30 minutes. Cooking and baking are considered "light" activities when it comes to

Table 4-1. Calories Burned by Doing Household Chores and Yard Work

Activity Category	Average Calories Burned/30 Minutes*
Light	0–90
Cooking/Baking	
Dusting	
Laundry	
Light carpentry	
Sweeping floors	
Washing dishes	
Moderate	90–130
Gardening	
Mowing with power mower	
Hedging/trimming lawn	
Raking leaves	
Scrubbing floors	
Carrying out trash	
Vacuuming floors	
Washing cars	
Washing windows	
Hard	Over 200
Digging earth	
Shoveling snow	
Heavy carpentry/home repair	

*Calories burned per 30 min are determined for an individual who weighs 150 pounds. Actual calories burned are slightly less for individuals who weigh under 150 pounds and are slightly more for individuals who weigh over 150 pounds. It is assumed that activities are done with moderate effort.

calorie burning; they burn 90–100 calories in 30 minutes. Walking is a "moderate" activity; when you walk for 30 minutes, you burn about 150 calories. Examples of a "hard" activity—one that requires more effort to complete and burns 200 calories or more in 30 minutes—would be shoveling snow, digging in the garden, or doing heavy home repair.

Though routine household tasks may not always be fun or rewarding, it is nice to know that when you do physical work around the house or in the yard it can contribute significantly to your overall health.

Being Active at Play

Leisure time at home is valuable time. We should all budget more time for leisure, even during the busiest periods in our lives. It's our opportunity to do things simply for the enjoyment of doing them. And if your leisure time is physically active, it has the added benefit of contributing to your good health and fitness. Table 4-2 identifies a variety of leisure activities, their calorie-burning potential, and the types of activity benefits they offer. Like work-related tasks, each leisure activity offers a

Table 4-2. Primary Activity Benefits of Sports and Leisure-Time Activities

Activity Category	Average Calories Burned/30 Minutes*	Types of Activity Benefits Burn Calories/ Strengthen Heart	Strengthen Muscles	Improve Balance/ Flexibility
Very Light	50–90			
Computer games, etc.				
Playing cards				
Reading				
Sewing/knitting				
Watching TV				
Light	90–120			
Billiards				✓
Bowling			✓	✓
Stationary cycling (5 mph)		✓	✓	
Golf (riding cart)			✓	✓
Stretching				✓
Walking/strolling (2 mph)		✓		
Wii Fit™ Yoga or Balance			✓	✓

Activity Category	Average Calories Burned/30 Minutes*	Types of Activity Benefits Burn Calories/ Strengthen Heart	Strengthen Muscles	Improve Balance/ Flexibility
Moderate	**120–190**			
Badminton		✓		✓
Brisk walking (>4 mph)		✓		✓
Calisthenics			✓	✓
Cycling (8–10 mph)		✓	✓	✓
Dance (ballroom)		✓	✓	✓
Fishing (walking and wading)		✓	✓	✓
Golf (walking/carrying clubs)		✓	✓	✓
Table tennis		✓		✓
Tennis (recreational)		✓	✓	✓
Volleyball		✓	✓	✓
Water exercise (aerobics)		✓	✓	✓
Wii Fit™ Running		✓	✓	
Hard	**200 or more**			
Cycling (>10 mph)		✓	✓	✓
Vigorous dance (aerobic, Zumba, square dance)		✓	✓	✓
Handball		✓	✓	
Jogging (>5 mph)		✓		
Swimming (moderate effort)		✓	✓	✓
Singles tennis (competitive)		✓	✓	✓
Weight lifting (hard effort)			✓	✓

*Calories burned in 30 min are determined for an individual who weighs 150 pounds. Actual calories burned are slightly less for individuals who weigh less than 150 pounds and are slightly more for individuals who weigh more than 150 pounds. It is assumed that activities are done with moderate effort.

unique set of benefits and can contribute to overall fitness in more than one way.

Notice that "very light" leisure activities require little movement, so the calories you burn and the activity benefits you gain from them are pretty small, so limit the amount of time you spend doing these activities. If you enjoy reading or watching TV, consider riding a stationary bicycle, walking on a treadmill, or marching in place at the same time. This way you can turn inactive leisure time into active time. Even if you're just sitting back watching TV, you can be active. On page 110, you'll find a series of stretching and strengthening exercises to do while you sit in an armchair. By doing these exercises, you can gain flexibility, increase strength and muscle tone, and rev up calorie burning—even while you watch your favorite program. At the very least, make it a practice to avoid sitting for a long period of time. Remember to get up every half hour or so and take a walk around your house, stretch for a few minutes, or do some light lifting and strengthening activities. These short bouts of activity that break up lengthy time spent sitting contribute significantly to your activity goals and improved health.

If you build some moderate activity into your leisure time, you see both health benefits and calorie-burning potential increase. A commitment to doing moderate activity may lead you to try new, fun forms of recreation or to resume leisure activities that you may have enjoyed in the past but haven't done recently.

Here are some fun ways to fit moderate activity into your day:

▶ Take a walk or hike with family or friends (you can do this in your neighborhood or go to a park for a special outing)
▶ Take your children (or grandchildren) to a neighborhood playground or outside in the yard and play
▶ Play a backyard game of badminton, volleyball, or croquet
▶ Play catch or shoot some baskets
▶ Play some favorite music and dance (children love this, too)
▶ If you have a backyard or neighborhood pool, get in and enjoy playing and moving in the water
▶ Try something new like yoga, aerobic dance, or Zumba by using a fitness DVD or video.

If you are planning on doing more vigorous exercise than you are accustomed to doing, be sure to discuss your exercise plans with your health care provider. By working with your provider, you can ensure the activity you plan to do is a safe option for you. More vigorous activities offer the advantage of burning more calories, but they also carry a greater risk of exercise-related injury than moderate activities. This is especially true if you try to do "hard" activities before you are physically ready. So, start slowly and—as you become more fit—gradually increase exercise intensity.

On the town

Another way to work activity into your leisure time is to make it part of everything you do when you're out on the town. Always be on the lookout for ways to build activity into inactive entertainment.

▶ When you go to movies, arrive early to buy your tickets, then take a walk until it's time to go in for the show.

▶ If you are out shopping, budget time to do some extra walking and window shopping.

▶ Find out about walking programs at your local mall. Plan your leisure-time shopping trips so that they match up with times when you can join other "mall walkers" in doing some uninterrupted, brisk walking before you shop.

▶ When you dine out, take advantage of opportunities to window shop or stroll in a park or along a waterfront area either while you wait to be seated or after you have finished your meal.

▶ If a restaurant is within walking distance of your home, don't touch those car keys! Make walking your mode of transportation.

▶ Save a few dollars and instead of using valet parking, park your own car and walk to restaurants and other establishments that offer valet parking.

▶ When you go to concerts, the theater, or other performances, arrive early and take a short walk to explore the area around the theater before the program begins. Always get up to stretch and walk during intermissions.

▶ Plan special, active outings with family and friends at parks or recreation areas.

▶ Try recreational activities that you may have enjoyed in the past, such as bowling or miniature golf.

▶ Consider trying ballroom, country, or other types of dance. Dancing can be a fun and vigorous way to increase activity during an evening out.

▶ Play golf on courses where you are allowed to walk and carry or pull your clubs.

▶ Go to a driving range or to batting cages where you can challenge yourself, sharpen your skills, and get some exercise at the same time.

▶ Join a tennis league.

- ▶ Take a class to learn yoga, tai chi, water aerobics, or other non-competitive forms of exercise and movement.
- ▶ Learn about popular areas for walking, cycling, or cross-country skiing in your city and try them out. Many cities have developed path or walkway systems where people can enjoy these activities in safe, park-like settings.
- ▶ Join a walking, cycling, or swimming club.
- ▶ Shoot some hoops at a local gym or on courts at a local park
- ▶ Do active volunteer work that you enjoy. Hospitals, youth programs, schools, museums, zoos, parks, and environmental associations often need and value the support of volunteers.

Leisure activities can take as much or as little time as you wish. Make it your goal to substitute "in-activities" with active leisure time. A good way to start is to keep track of how much time you spend sitting and being inactive during your free time each day. Then choose enjoyable, active alternatives to fill that time (Figure 4-1). In this way, you don't have to make time for activity; you can simply put the time you have to active, healthy use.

Figure 4-1. Daily Activity Evaluation

| | | TYPE OF ACTIVITY | |
| | | Active Alternative | |
	Inactive (minutes)	Work (minutes)	Leisure (minutes)
Morning 6:00 a.m. – 12:00 p.m.			
Afternoon 12:00 p.m. – 6:00 p.m.			
Evening 6:00 p.m. – 11:00 p.m.			
Nighttime Sleep from _____ to _____			

Being Active on the Job

Even in this age of economy, efficiency, and labor-saving devices, most American workers feel very pressed for time. With long commutes and constant connection to work through mobile devices and other demands that extend the workday, personal time is shrinking. And worse yet, for many, the typical day at work has become so inactive that it actually can be harmful to your health. A number of studies completed over the past 40 years have shown that people who are inactive at work have higher death rates than people who work in physically active jobs. Studies have also associated physical inactivity with a substantial number of deaths due to type 2 diabetes and related conditions. So, it is important to examine your typical workday and look at how active or inactive it is.

Table 4-3 offers examples of some physically active and some physically inactive jobs. Notice that the active jobs require people to do a fair amount of walking, as well as some work that requires muscle strength such as lifting, pulling, or pushing objects. Inactive jobs involve a lot of sitting and very little movement. If your work requires you to do a lot of sitting or to be very inactive for long periods of time, it is especially important for you to find ways to build activity breaks into your day.

Table 4-3. Examples of Physically Active vs. Physically Inactive Jobs

PHYSICALLY ACTIVE JOBS (Moderate)	PHYSICALLY INACTIVE JOBS
Carpenter/painter	Bank teller
Chef	Clerical worker
Farmer	Computer programmer
House cleaner	General office work
Nurse	Driver (bus, cab, truck, etc.)
Store clerk	Machinist
Tailor	Sales
Teacher	Telemarketer
Waitress	Writer

PHYSICALLY ACTIVE JOBS (Heavy)
Landscape/yard worker
Industrial worker

However, even if your job is fairly physically active, you can benefit from activity breaks to do some stretching and relieve muscle tension.

How to increase activity at work

Let's look at how you can build activity into your workday without taking time away from your responsibilities. First and foremost, find opportunities to do small amounts of activity throughout the day. This basic principle will help you to successfully become more active at work. Here are some examples of ways to squeeze activity into your workday:

- ▶ Get up 10 or 15 minutes earlier than usual and spend this time doing some activity before work. Take your dog for a walk or spend the extra minutes walking on the way into your office. Or do some stretching and light calisthenics after your morning shower, such as the Stretch and Strengthen Routine in chapter 8.
- ▶ If you're in the habit of grabbing a fast food meal on your commute, don't use the drive-through window: Park your car and walk into the restaurant—and always make the healthiest possible food choices!
- ▶ If safe to do so, park your car at a distant part of the office parking lot so that you can increase the amount of walking you do on your way in.
- ▶ If you use public transportation, get off a stop or two early and walk to your final destination.
- ▶ Use stairs instead of the elevator or escalator. If need be, take the elevator part of the way and the stairs the rest of the way, then gradually increase the number of floors you climb as you become more fit.
- ▶ If you go out for lunch, walk to your destination.
- ▶ Before you begin your commute home, take a walk. You may manage to miss the traffic rush and still get home at the usual time.
- ▶ When you have to work at your desk for an extended period of time, build short breaks into your day. For example:
  - ▶ Do a series of seated stretches (see chapter 8)

- Do a few easy strengthening activities at your desk (see chapter 8). Consider keeping some small hand-held and/or ankle weights or an exercise band in a desk drawer.
- Get up and take a quick walk around your office or go to the water fountain, mail drop, or copy machine.
- Use a speakerphone or a mobile phone so that you can get up and pace around your office during phone calls.
- Stand up or do some chair exercises (chapter 8) during phone calls.
- Spend part of your break taking a walk.

As you can see, these suggestions require very little time, and you can do many of them while you work. For example, do a few foot and toe stretches while you are at your computer, or a few seated knee extensions while sitting in a meeting. Short activity sessions that allow you to leave your work for a few minutes can be very beneficial and are usually well justified. When you return, you will be re-energized, more focused, more productive, and less tense than before the activity session.

It is not necessary to have special exercise equipment at work to increase your daily activity. Just plan ahead a little. If you decide to take short walks or climb stairs as part of your fitness routine, be sure to wear comfortable and supportive shoes. If you plan to take fairly long walks during lunch or after work, keep a good pair of walking shoes and athletic socks in your office to change into for your walk. Having access to good shoes will keep you comfortable as well as minimize the risk of injury to your feet from ill-fitting shoes—an important consideration if you have neuropathy or poor circulation in your feet. You may also decide to keep an exercise band or a pair of light weights in your desk drawer; you can use them to add effort to light calisthenics or strengthening activities you do at your desk. A bottle of water works nicely as a dumbbell for increasing resistance as well.

As always, the overall goal is to keep it simple and do small amounts of activity frequently throughout the workday. Even if you do just 5 minutes of activity each hour during an 8-hour workday and walk for 20 minutes during your lunch break, you will accumulate 60 minutes of physical activity—that's good progress toward reaching a goal of doing 150 minutes (or more) of weekly activity!

On the road

Work-related travel can really disrupt your physical activity routine, but luckily, there are ways to meet the challenge. Once again the basic principle of doing small amounts of activity frequently throughout the day will help you stay physically active when you're on the road. Here are some suggestions for fitting in activity on travel days:

When you travel by air:

▶ budget time to do some extra walking in airports, for example walk instead of using a moving walkway;

▶ if you have a carry-on bag, think about actively using your muscles as you pull, push, and lift it on your way through the airport;

▶ do some stretches on the airplane or while you wait for your flight (see the seated stretches on pages 110–113);

▶ during a long flight, get up and move periodically, and if you can find some space at the back of the plane, do some standing stretches (see page 126).

When you travel by car:

▶ make time to get out of your car every few hours and walk for 5 or 10 minutes;

▶ stretch for a few minutes whenever you stop to buy gas;

▶ when you stop for meals, always get out of your car; walk for 10 minutes either before or after you eat.

When you stay out of town:

▶ take advantage of downtime to do some stretching and strengthening activities in your hotel room (see page 110), and, if you wish, pack light weights or an exercise band to use in your fitness routine;

▶ march in place while you watch TV or turn on some music and dance;

▶ if your hotel has an exercise facility or pool, use it. Walk on a treadmill, ride a stationary bike while you watch the evening news, swim, or lift weights;

> ▶ walk and explore the city you are visiting on foot, or walk to meetings or to nearby restaurants.

It's true that travel can be unpredictable and tiring. As a result, your focus may simply be on getting to your destination and home again, rather than on keeping up with your daily physical activity. But if you create a healthy travel plan and have it in place before you leave on your trip, this will help you stay on track with your exercise plan as well as other health goals. And if you exercise, you may find it makes travel less tiring and more enjoyable. As part of your travel plan, try to identify certain things:

> ▶ Ways to fit small amounts of activity into your day. Any amount of movement helps, but aim to do at least one, 10-minute session of continuous activity. Remind yourself that even when you feel fatigued, moderate physical activity can energize you.
> ▶ Healthy foods. Don't be a victim of unhealthy meals and snacks in airports or on the road. Remember that the availability of food on flights is limited, so the best option is to bring along your own meals and snacks.
> ▶ Ways to drink plenty of fluids and maintain proper hydration.
> ▶ The diabetes supplies that you will need to have with you (meter, strips, medications, and a treatment for hypoglycemia).

When you take steps to stay active and healthy when you travel, you will feel good, be able to enjoy your travels, and will be more focused and productive throughout the day.

Really Run Those Errands!

Most Americans spend a lot of time out-and-about around town running errands, doing household shopping, or going to appointments. Unfortunately, because of city sprawl, we are likely to spend more time driving and parking our cars than burning calories when we are out running errands. Few of us have the option of taking care of errands in a neighborhood or tightly spaced downtown area as we did in the past, so we need to find ways to build activity back into our lives when we are out-and-about.

Two birds with one stone

You probably feel rushed when you're running errands or taking care of appointments and other personal business and the thought of making these errands *more* active is tiring in and of itself. However, with some planning ahead and willingness to change your usual habits, it is possible to fit in quick activity sessions during these times and accomplish two things at once. The benefit is noticeably higher activity levels, improved health, and reduced feelings of stress, strain, and fatigue when you return home.

So, let's consider strategies for building activity into the routine task of running errands and taking care of personal business.

- ▶ Have your trip planned and organized before you start out.
  - ▶ Determine the most efficient route for driving in order to minimize the amount of time you spend sitting in your car.
  - ▶ If possible, schedule appointments and run errands when you know that traffic and crowds are the lightest. This will help prevent a sense of urgency, which can be a big barrier to fitting in activity.
  - ▶ Organize your trip so that you cluster errands together if they are near each other. Then park your car once and walk between stops.
- ▶ Make an effort to walk whenever possible.
  - ▶ If safe to do so, park your car at the far end of parking lots so that you increase the amount of walking you do on your way into stores and businesses.
  - ▶ Walk between errands when the stores and businesses you need to visit are close to one another.
  - ▶ If you have errands to do at a mall, schedule your day so that you do them in the morning. Then arrive 30 minutes before the stores open and do some brisk walking before you start shopping.
- ▶ Take stairs instead of escalators and elevators.
- ▶ Avoid using drive-through windows. Always get out of your car and walk into businesses that offer drive-through options, such as banks, restaurants, and dry cleaners.

- ▶ If you use public transportation, get off a stop or two away from your final destination and walk the added distance.
- ▶ Make an effort to pick up the pace a bit and walk briskly!
- ▶ Use your own muscles to do work.
  - ▷ Carry your own groceries and shopping bags.
  - ▷ When you have the option, avoid using doors that open automatically. Instead, push or pull doors open yourself.
- ▶ If you are standing and waiting in a line, do some arm, shoulder, or neck stretches (see page 126).
- ▶ If you are sitting and waiting, do a few chair exercises or stretches (see page 110).

You may not be able to say you literally "ran" those errands, but you certainly picked up the pace and did them in an active way! And that's the important thing to remember: If you want to make activity and improved health and fitness a part of your life forever, it can be as simple as doing everything—from housework to play to travel—in a more active way. Decide to leave the car and walk when you can. Decide to climb stairs instead of riding escalators and elevators. Decide to carry your own packages and open a door. You don't have to carry all the groceries or climb every flight; you just have to start one step—or one push, pull, or lift—at a time.

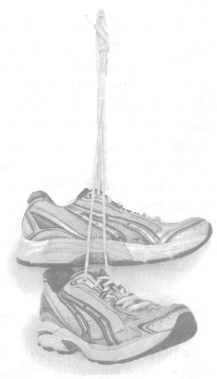

Chapter 5

KEEP GOING: ACTIVITY FOR A LIFETIME

Setting Goals for a Lifetime of Physical Activity

Every New Year's Day, countless people resolve to lose weight and get in shape—and they want to do it fast! The phones in fitness centers ring off the hook, new members join, and members who haven't been to the gym in months start to show up. The exercise classes are full and all the workout equipment is in use at peak times of the day. For a while, people exercise like crazy, but, within a month or two, many begin to drop out and things slow down to the normal pace. Within 3–6 months, only half of the people who started to exercise will continue to stick with it. This same scenario plays out in weight loss or weight management centers as well. The phones ring and people join programs and start dieting to lose those extra pounds quickly! However, before long, many dieters get tired of feeling hungry and restricted in their eating and are frustrated when they fail to shed all the weight they had hoped to lose in an impossibly short amount of time. So they quit.

These people were looking for a quick fix rather than making a commitment to a long-term lifestyle change. Unfortunately, the end result of quick-fix thinking is typically repeated failure, frustration, and little progress toward achieving better health and fitness. Quick-fix thinking just doesn't support the reality of becoming more physically active for lifelong health and well-being. Consider this: Within two weeks of stopping a physical activity program, health benefits begin to disappear. Within three months of stopping, health gains from previous exercise training disappear altogether. So, it pays to think long-term about establishing a physical activity habit that will help you achieve a lifetime of good health and physical fitness.

Develop a fitness habit

Building moderate amounts of physical activity into your lifestyle is an important first step toward healthy, active living. Congratulations! If you've started implementing some of the things we've discussed so far, you're well on your way. Now it's time to go a step further and make a lifelong commitment. This means forming a physical activity habit. Developing this habit is an ongoing process that involves goal setting as well as a number of other tactics. For long-term success:

▶ Think of goal setting as an ongoing process and as a skill you can develop. Continuously evaluate and adjust your physical activity goals to ensure they are helping you to make gradual progress toward becoming more active. Remain flexible and willing to adjust your goals as needed.

▶ For the first 3–4 months of building more activity into your weekly routine, set an activity goal each week. At the end of the week, consider how you did, what went well, and what challenges or barriers got in the way. Based on your experience, adjust your goal(s) as needed until you devise a plan that results in success reaching your goal.

▶ Keep your goals challenging and motivating, yet realistic. Remember that if they are too easy to reach, your goals may not challenge you enough to keep you motivated. If your goals are too difficult to achieve, you may become frustrated and discouraged and give up.

▶ At challenging times, when it is difficult to fit activity in, be flexible and try different things. Be open to adapting and resetting your goals at an easier level for a while.

▶ Update and change your self-contract to reflect your modified goals.

▶ Every once in a while, change the rewards you give yourself so that they continue to be meaningful and to reinforce your exercise habit.

Once you establish a firm habit of doing things in a physically active way each day, you will have built a solid fitness foundation. This will go a long way toward helping you remain physically active, even at times when life throws you a curve.

Now you are ready to take the next step: to further increase the amount of physical activity you do. With this next step, you can gain additional health benefits and a higher level of fitness.

What's the next step?

As you continue to get in shape, fitness and health experts recommend gradually increasing your amount of physical activity until you are able to accrue at least 150 minutes (2 1/2 hours) of weekly activity, the goal suggested by the U.S. Physical Activity Guidelines. As a starting point, each activity session should include at least 10 minutes of nonstop activity. If you are already at this level, gradually start to add some time to your total minutes of daily activity. You may decide to work toward doing at least three 10-minute sessions of activity per day. Alternatively, you may decide to do fewer activity sessions but have each one last for a longer amount of time. For example, you may choose to do one, 30-minute or two, 15-minute sessions of activity for a daily total of 30 minutes.

Remember, for optimal glucose lowering, routinely include physical activity in your schedule and go no more than two consecutive days without doing any exercise.

It is possible to reach an even higher level of fitness and greater health benefits by continuing to gradually increase the amount of activity you do. You may even get to a point where you'd like to add a fitness class or other forms of structured exercise to your routine of moderate lifestyle activity. Remember, the progress you make and how quickly you make it is based on your personal fitness goals. It is completely up to you!

Working toward higher activity goals

Once you are in the habit of routinely doing moderate activity on most days and you are feeling good doing it, you are ready to further increase your physical activity level. Now you can start to:
1. Gradually increase your total minutes of daily and weekly activity.
2. Increase how long you exercise at one time—gradually adding a minute or two on to your sessions.

The rate at which you increase activity time depends a lot on how you feel, but most experts recommend simply increasing the amount of moderate activity that you do by a minute or two each day.

Here is an example. Let's say that you are currently able to walk for 15 minutes comfortably without stopping and you do this two times a day—during your lunch break, and in the evening. Your goal is to gradually increase the amount of time that you walk in the evening. You eventually want to walk continuously for 30 minutes each evening in order to achieve a daily total of 45 minutes of walking. So, the first thing you do is add 1 minute onto your evening walk for a total of 16 minutes during this session. You keep your midday walk at 15 minutes due to time limitations during the lunch hour. If the longer evening walk goes well and you feel comfortable with the 1-minute increase, you are probably ready to add another minute or two onto your total walking time. The next day you may decide to walk for 18 minutes in the evening. As a result, you will accumulate a daily total of 33 minutes of walking. That's a 10% increase in exercise in just a few days, and that's good progress! Continue adding a minute or two onto your daily activity time as you're ready and soon you'll be exercising at least 45 minutes each day.

Remember that you should not feel pain, discomfort, or too much fatigue as you increase the amount of activity you do. You don't want injuries or setbacks at this point, so be careful not to do too much too fast. If you're injured, it's hard to do much exercise at all. In fact, consider talking to your health care provider before you significantly increase your physical activity routine. Be certain to ask questions and discuss concerns you have about exercising with pre-diabetes, diabetes, or other health-related issues. Slow, steady, and sensible progress is healthy progress.

What about structured exercise?

After you become comfortable with increased levels of daily physical activity, you may be so happy about how you feel and look that you decide to add some structured exercise to your fitness routine. This step, though definitely a good move in terms of improving fitness and gaining health benefits, is not something you *must* do. But if you do decide to take part in structured exercise, consider consulting your health care provider beforehand, especially if you will be doing new types of activity or more vigorous activities than before. This is particularly important if you have certain health conditions. Table 5-1 is a pre-exercise health assessment that helps you identify reasons for consulting your health care team before beginning a structured or vigorous exercise program.

Adding structured exercise can improve your physical fitness to a degree that will allow you to do the things you want to do in daily life and to feel healthy and vigorous while doing them. However, before you get to this point, it might be helpful to understand what we really mean when we talk about "physical fitness." Basically, physical fitness is made up of four components.

1. Cardiorespiratory Endurance

This reflects the ability of the heart, lungs, and circulatory system to efficiently supply oxygen throughout the body. Cardiorespiratory endurance is measured by your ability to do aerobic exercise—activity that requires continuous, rhythmic use of large muscles—at a moderate-to-vigorous level (for example, to walk briskly for one mile).

2. Body Composition

Body composition goes a step beyond simply stating your weight in pounds; it tells you what percentage of your body is lean muscle mass and what percentage is fat. For example, a football player may seem to be overweight when he tips the scales at 250 pounds, but most of that may

Table 5-1. Good Reasons to Consult Your Physician before Beginning Exercise

Assess your health by putting a check next to all true statements.

History

You have had

_____ a heart attack

_____ heart surgery (bypass, angioplasty, pacemaker, valve repair, etc.)

_____ cardiac catheterization

_____ defibrillator/rhythm disturbance

_____ heart valve disease

_____ heart failure

_____ heart transplantation

_____ congenital heart condition

_____ a stroke

_____ peripheral artery disease

Symptoms

_____ You experience chest discomfort with exertion

_____ You experience unreasonable breathlessness

_____ You experience dizziness, fainting, or blackouts

_____ You take heart medications

> *If you marked any of these statements in this section, consult your physician or other appropriate health care provider before beginning a new exercise program.*

Other health issues

_____ You have diabetes

_____ You have specific diabetes complications including neuropathy/autonomic neuropathy, retinopathy, or nephropathy/renal failure

_____ You have asthma or other lung disease

_____ You have burning or cramping sensation in your lower legs when walking a short distance

_____ You have musculoskeletal problems that limit your physical activity

_____ You have concerns about the safety of exercise

_____ You take prescription medications

_____ You are pregnant

Cardiovascular Risk Factors

_____ You are over 40 years (and have diabetes)

_____ You are over 30 years and you have had diabetes for over 10 years

_____ You smoke or you quit smoking within the previous 6 months

_____ Your blood pressure is over 140/90 mm Hg

_____ You do not know your blood pressure

_____ You take blood pressure medications

_____ Your blood cholesterol is over 200 mg/dl

_____ You do not know your cholesterol level

_____ You have a close blood relative who had a heart attack or heart surgery before age 55 (father or brother) or age 65 (mother or sister)

_____ You are physically inactive (you do less than 30 minutes of physical activity on at least 3 days per week)

_____ You are 20 pounds or more overweight

> *If you marked any of these statements in this section, consult your physician or other appropriate health care provider before beginning a new exercise program.*

If you marked any of these statements in this section, consult your physician or other appropriate health care provider before beginning a new exercise program

Adapted from: American College of Sports Medicine and American Heart Association. ACSM/AHA Joint Position Statement: Recommendations for cardiovascular screening, staffing, and emergency policies at health/fitness facilities. *Med Sci Sports Exer:* 1012.

American College of Sports Medicine, American Diabetes Association. Joint position statement: Exercise and type 2 diabetes. *Diabetes Care* 33; c147–c167.

be muscle and not fat. Having a high percentage of body fat, not just being overweight, increases health risks.

3. Muscular Strength and Endurance

This reflects your ability to do a given amount of muscular work over a period of time. For example, a measure of your strength and endurance would be how many bicep curls you could do using a 5-pound weight while maintaining good form.

4. Flexibility

This component measures your ability to move your joints freely and without pain through a full range of motion. For example, rotating your shoulder joint a full 90 degrees without pain reflects excellent range of motion for that joint. Depending on the type of structured exercise you do, it should allow you to maintain or to gradually improve one or more of these physical fitness components. Let's look at how to do this, using a guide called the FITT Principle.

Improve Your FITTness

The FITT Principle sets exercise goals for adults who are trying to improve their health and physical fitness. Developed by experts in the field, the FITT Principle provides guidelines on exercise:

Frequency—how many times to exercise each week
Intensity—how vigorously or with how much effort to do an exercise
Time—how long to spend doing an exercise
Type—the kind of exercise to do

Using the FITT Principle as our guide, let's look at recommended exercise goals for improving each of the components of physical fitness.

Cardiorespiratory fitness

Improving cardiorespiratory fitness not only increases oxygen supply throughout the body, it can also improve risk factors for heart and circulatory diseases. To improve cardiorespiratory fitness, follow the FITT Principle recommendations.

Frequency

Exercise three to five times per week with no more than two day in a row between exercise sessions.

Intensity

Think moderate. You should exercise at 50–70% of the maximal heart rate for your age-group (see Table 5-2). Your RPE (rating of perceived exertion) should be in the 12–14 range (see Figure 3-1, page 37), and you should be able to talk while you exercise. If you are too out of breath to pass the "talk test," slow down!

Table 5-2. Determining Target Heart Rate for Exercise

	Example
1. Subtract your age from 220 to determine your age-predicted maximal heart rate (HRmax)	220 – 50 = 170
2. Multiply your HRmax by 50% and by 70% to determine your target heart rate zone for exercise in beats per minute	
HRmax x 0.50 = bottom of target zone	170 x .50 = 85
HRmax x 0.70 = top of target zone	170 x .70 = 119
3. Divide your target zone numbers (beats per minute) by 6 to determine your 10-second (sec) pulse count	
Bottom of target zone (lower pulse count number ÷6)	85÷6 =14.1(14)
Top of target zone (upper pulse count number ÷6)	119 ÷6 =19.8(20)
4. Your target heart rate range for aerobic exercise is between your bottom and top target zone and is measured by 10-second pulse count	85–119 beats/min 14–20 beats/10 sec

Caution! *For exercise safety,* consider seeing your physician before using a target heart rate range calculated by using this formula. This will assure that the range you calculate is correct for you. Certain heart conditions as well as heart and blood pressure medications can cause target heart rate ranges for exercise to differ from calculated values.

Time

Build up toward doing 20–60 minutes of exercise, completed in either one session of continuous activity or through several shorter sessions, each lasting at least 10 minutes.

Type

Perform aerobic activities that use large muscle groups in a rhythmic, continuous way (see Table 5-3).

Body weight and body composition

If you have been struggling to lose a few pounds or if you've noticed an extra inch or two that you can pinch, you're not alone. Our society as a whole has been getting heavier. Carrying extra pounds, especially around your midsection, increases the risk of developing diabetes, heart disease, and high blood pressure, as well as other chronic diseases. When you have pre-diabetes or type 2 diabetes, you already run a higher risk

Table 5-3. Aerobic Exercise: What Counts?

Forms of Aerobic Exercise	Calories Burned/30 Min*
Aerobic dance/group dance†	205
Dance general (e.g., ballroom)	153
Bicycling/cycling	
12–14 mph	205
Leisurely	136
Cross-country skiing	272
Hiking	204
Jogging/running†	239
Rope skipping†	341
Rowing	239
Skating	239
Stair climbing†	204
Swimming	273
Water exercise	136
Walking	119

*Calories burned per 30 min are determined for an individual who weighs 150 pounds. Actual calories burned are slightly less for individuals who weigh under 150 pounds and are slightly more for individuals who weigh over 150 pounds. It is assumed that activities are done with moderate effort.

†Many of these activities are high impact. Check with your physician, especially if you have diabetes complications, to assure that these are safe options for you.

Ainsworth, B.A., Haskell, W.L., Leon, A.S., et al. Compendium of physical activities: classification of energy costs of human physical activities. *Med Sci Sports Exer* 25:71–80.

for heart disease and high blood pressure. Fortunately, moderate weight loss of just 10 or 20 pounds can help reduce blood glucose levels and improve your body's sensitivity to insulin, help reduce blood pressure, and improve cardiovascular risk factors.

While healthy eating and keeping calories in check are important to success with any weightloss program, physical activity is essential too. Exercise helps build and maintain lean muscle while it burns extra body fat as fuel. Regular exercise also helps prevent further weight gain and keeps pounds off once they are lost. To improve your body weight and composition, follow these FITT Principle recommendations.

Frequency

Exercise five to seven times per week. Being active most every day is an optimal goal.

Intensity

Once again, think moderate. You should exercise at 50–60% of the maximal heart rate for your age group (see Table 5-2). The RPE (rating of perceived exertion) should be in the 12–14 range (see Figure 3-1, page 34). And you should be able to talk while you exercise. If you are too out of breath to pass the "talk test"—slow down!

Time

Aim to do *at least* 250 minutes of physical activity per week. Studies have shown that people who exercise for longer amounts of time—between 200 and 300 minutes (about 3 1/2 to 5 hours) per week, have the best success with losing weight and keeping pounds off long-term.

Type

Aerobic activity is your best choice for burning calories and supporting weight loss (see Table 5-3). Doing strength training or resistance exercises 2–3 times per week will help maintain or increase lean muscle.

Additional considerations for weight loss and maintenance

When you are exercising for weight control, your main goal is to burn calories. Aerobic exercise, the type that uses large muscles repetitively and continuously, is the best when it comes to burning calories and reducing body fat. At first, try to burn *at least* 1,000 calories per week. That sounds like a lot, but that's just around 150 extra calories per day. Experts generally agree that the safest way to reach this goal is to keep exercise intensity at a comfortable and moderate level and to exercise for the amount of time it takes to tally up 1,000 calories burned. Usually, this requires about 150 minutes of activity per week. Here are a few ways to accumulate this amount:

▶ Exercise 7 days per week and do enough activity to burn 150 calories each day (about 20–25 minutes per day).

- Exercise 4 days per week and do enough activity on each of those days to burn 250 calories (about 35–40 minutes per day).
- Exercise 3 days per week and do enough activity on each of those days to burn about 300 calories (about 50 minutes per day).

The bottom line is that it is better to do longer amounts of moderate activity and be comfortable than to do hard, fast, intense exercise that can be uncomfortable and lead to muscle pain, soreness, or injury.

3,500: The Magic Number

What makes the number 3,500 so special? That's the number of calories you need to burn to lose 1 pound of body fat. If you burn 500 calories more than you take in every day for one week, you should lose about 1 pound in that week. However, weight loss doesn't always occur at a steady rate. You may lose weight quickly and easily at first but find that the pounds come off more slowly over time. In part, that is because you lose extra body water along with fat at first. As you continue to lose weight, changes occur in your body as a result of weight loss. For example, you carrying around fewer extra pounds (a good thing), but this means you need fewer calories to support daily functions and movement. So, as you continue your weight loss efforts, you may find it necessary to periodically re-evaluate your progress and either reduce your calorie intake further or increase your amount of physical activity. Aiming for a 1–2 pound per week weight loss is realistic and safe for most people. Just think, if you burn 500 calories more than you take in every day for a year, and lose about a pound per week, that's a weight loss of 52 pounds a year.

Once you have reached a goal of burning 1,000 more calories or doing 150 additional minutes of activity per week, continue building on to this foundation. Next, aim to burn 2,000 additional calories per week. This can usually be accomplished by adding 200–300 minutes more to your weekly exercise time (about 30–45 minutes per day). This amount of activity and level of calorie burning has been shown to help keep extra weight off once it has been lost. If adding as much as 200–300 minutes seems like a lot, take heart; once you get into a solid physical activity

Figure 5-1. Landmarks for Finding Your Pulse Count

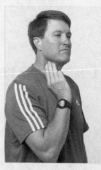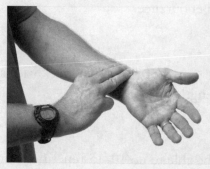

▶ Using your middle and index fingers, locate your pulse at the side of your neck or base of your wrist (press down only lightly at the site)

▶ Count the number of beats that you feel in 10 seconds—begin counting with the first beat you feel and count 0,1,2,3... until 10 seconds is up.

▶ Multiply your 10-second pulse count by 6 to determine your heart rate in beats per minute.

habit, lose some extra pounds, and become more fit, it won't seem like that much.

Muscle strength and endurance

We need muscle strength every day to do things like pushing the vacuum cleaner or lawn mower or lifting a child or grandchild into our arms. When our muscles are strong, we are able to work and play and do all the things we want to do each day without giving it a second thought. Maintaining good muscle strength and endurance allows us to function independently and at an optimal level as we age.

The types of exercises that help keep muscles strong are called resistance or strength training activities. They include calisthenics, weight lifting, core stability training, and other exercises that strengthen specific muscle groups. You don't need special equipment to do strengthening exercises. However, if you choose to use weight training equipment in a fitness center or purchase equipment for home use, be certain to have a trained fitness professional show you how to use the equipment safely and correctly. The strengthening exercises included in chapter 8, in the section titled *Sit, Stretch, and Strengthen*, are some that you may wish to do at home or even in your office during the work day. Follow the FITT

Principle guidelines for these and other exercises to increase muscle strength and endurance.

Frequency

Perform exercises 2 or 3 days per week with at least 2 days (48 hours) between strength training sessions.

Intensity

You should be able to do 10–15 repetitions of an exercise with good form before you become too tired. If you can easily do more repetitions than this, slightly increase the amount of weight or resistance that you work against. If you have difficulty doing this many repetitions, start with fewer repetitions (4–6) and gradually increase the number that you do.

Time

Strength and endurance exercises generally aren't timed like aerobic exercises. Instead, they're often based on repetitions and sets of repetitions. Include 8–10 different exercises that target major muscles of the body including arm, shoulder, chest, abdominal, leg, and lower back muscles. Plan to do 2–4 sets (series of repetitions) of each exercise. A balanced routine usually takes 20–30 minutes to complete.

Type

Resistance exercises include: calisthenics, weight lifting, activities that use exercise bands, medicine or stability balls, or water exercise.

Additional considerations for muscle strength and endurance

Remember these safety tips when you do resistance exercises or calisthenics:

- ▶ Start slowly and gradually build up repetitions, amount of resistance, and exercise sets as you get stronger
- ▶ Do slow, steady, and controlled movements—avoid jerking or straining
- ▶ Position your body properly
- ▶ Focus on breathing throughout the exercise—avoid holding your breath

- ▶ Stop any exercise that causes pain—cut back if you feel soreness or stiffness
- ▶ Keep it comfortable

Stretching and flexibility

Some exercisers overlook stretching and flexibility exercises because they don't seem like real exercise. However, stretching is a vital part of a balanced fitness routine. It helps you maintain the ability to move your joints freely and without pain through a good range of motion. The FITT guidelines for stretching that can help you achieve and maintain optimal flexibility and range of motion are:

Frequency

Perform stretches 2 or 3 days per week, as well as part of any warm-up or cool-down period of exercising.

Intensity

Don't overdo it! Stretch just to the point where you feel mild tension or discomfort. It's OK to feel a slight pull, but not pain. If you feel pain, release your stretch.

Type

Try to target your major joints and muscle groups, including the arms, shoulders, chest, abdominals, lower back, hips, knees, ankles, and leg muscles.

Time

Each stretch should last for 5–15 seconds and should be repeated 2–4 times.

Additional considerations for stretching and flexibility

When you stretch, remember these tips for comfort and safety:
- ▶ Stretching exercises are best to do when your muscles are warm. Stretch at the end of the warm-up or as part of the cool-down at the end of an exercise session.

- ▶ Ease off if you feel pain or more than mild discomfort while stretching
- ▶ Avoid bobbing, bouncing, or straining
- ▶ Breathe naturally and slowly while you stretch

Putting It All Together

With these goals and guidelines in mind, it's time to create your own personal exercise routine. Remember, all the activities that you do each day provide a solid foundation on which to build an exercise routine. It is important to continue to include these unstructured activities in your day even as you introduce, and then increase, planned exercise.

Before you begin to exercise, take time to organize the activities you plan to do into a safe and enjoyable routine. Any well-planned exercise session will include three components:

1. **Warm-up.** The warm-up is intended to prepare your muscles, joints, heart, and lungs for more vigorous activity. Start with 5–10 minutes of light or easy aerobic activity, such as low-intensity walking or cycling, followed by 5–10 minutes of stretching. Warm-up activities should focus on muscle groups that you plan to use during more vigorous exercise.

2. **Aerobic Phase.** This phase of an exercise session should include 20–60 minutes of aerobic activity (Table 5-3). During the aerobic phase, maintain your desired exercise intensity using target heart rate (Table 5-2), RPE (page 65), and/or the "talk test" (page 66) as guides. As an option you may do shorter sessions throughout the day, each lasting at least 10 minutes.

3. **Cool-down.** The purpose of the first part of a cool-down is to gradually bring your heart rate down to its pre-exercise level. It should include 5–10 minutes of light or easy aerobic activity. Follow the aerobic part of your cool-down with some calisthenics, weight lifting, or strengthening exercises. Finish up with some stretching.

If you choose to do strengthening exercises, such as weight lifting, on alternate days when you don't do aerobic exercise, it is important to include a warm-up and cool-down as part of your exercise session.

Go at your own pace

If you feel ready to plan and begin an individualized exercise routine, consider having a conversation with your health care provider to get their OK and ensure your plan is the best option for you. You may also want to do a simple physical fitness self-assessment (see Appendix 2, *Simple Physical Fitness Self-Assessment* on page 141). This will help you identify your beginning fitness level and will help you gauge your progress as you get in better shape.

Whatever your personal goals and expectations are at this point, it pays to remember the tale of the tortoise and the hare. When it comes

Table 5-4. Summary of Goals: Activity for Health, Exercise for Fitness, and Activity for Weight Management

	Activity for Health	Exercise for Fitness	Activity for Weight Management
Frequency	Frequently throughout the day, work toward doing 10-minute sessions	3–5 days per week*	5–7 days per week*
Intensity	"Moderate" "talk test"	"Moderate to vigorous" (measure using heart rate = 50–70% age predicted or RPE = 12–15 (somewhat hard–hard)	"Moderate" Or an RPE = 12–14 (somewhat hard)
Time	30 minutes of activity on most days; total at least 150 min. (2 ½ hours) per week	20–60 minutes of moderate–vigorous exercise to total at least 150 min. (2 ½ hours)	45–60 minutes of activity on most days to total 300 minutes (5 hours) per week
	time can be accumulated through shorter, 10-minute sessions done throughout the day		
Type	Moderate lifestyle activity/general muscle movement	Aerobic exercise plus muscle strengthening and stretching	Aerobic exercise plus muscle strengthening and stretching and lifestyle activity

*Aim for no more than 2 consecutive days between exercise bouts to maximize improvement in insulin action and blood glucose control.

to doing physical activity, whether it is informal daily activity or planned exercise, slow, steady progress leads to success. When you accept the idea that becoming active and physically fit is a gradual process that takes time and commitment, you will achieve—and possibly even exceed— your own goals and expectations. You will enjoy the process of being active and fit and living vigorously. However, if unrealistic goals and expectations lead you to do too much too fast, you will be at risk of experiencing setbacks and burnout, both of which can contribute to lack of progress and failure to succeed in the long run. Start slow and reward your steady progress. The prize at the end of the road is better health, a higher level of fitness, a greater sense of well-being, and an "I can do it" outlook.

Tailoring Your Management Plan

This is probably a good point to step back and take a look, once again, at why we're doing all of this activity in the first place. Physical activity is an important part of staying healthy with pre-diabetes or diabetes and should be incorporated into a total plan for either preventing or managing diabetes. That means the activity you do and other steps you take to manage your condition—including healthy eating, taking medications, staying positive, managing stress, and blood glucose monitoring—should complement one another. Let's look at how monitoring your glucose and A1c can help you learn how to fit activity into your diabetes or pre-diabetes plan so that you can achieve the best possible blood glucose results.

When preventing diabetes

If you have been told you have pre-diabetes, be sure to regularly followup with your health care provider. You should get checked for type 2 diabetes every one or two years. Lifestyle changes that you make are vital for preventing or delaying onset of diabetes. Remember, these include: losing a modest amount of weight—10 to 20 pounds for most people— getting 150 minutes (2 1/2 hours) of physical activity per week, and following a healthy, low-fat eating pattern.

When managing diabetes

What should your blood glucose levels be? Ideally, they should be in a goal range that you and your health care provider decide is best for you. The risk of developing diabetes complications is greatly reduced when blood glucose levels are kept as close to normal as possible and your A1C is < 7%. Everyone should determine their own target ranges with their health care team, but in general, desirable target ranges are:

▶ 70–130 mg/dl pre-meal
▶ 100–140 mg/dl at bedtime
▶ 180 mg/dl or less 1–2 hours after a meal

Reaching and keeping your blood glucose levels in these ranges once you start to build regular physical activity into your routine can take some fine-tuning of your diabetes plan. You may hit on just the right balance immediately, or it may take some time to adjust your plan to accommodate your more active lifestyle.

Blood glucose monitoring and decision making

As you add physical activity to your daily routine, some extra blood glucose testing before and after you exercise can help you gain understanding of how physical activity affects your glucose level. Extra monitoring can also help you make informed decisions about adjusting your diabetes plan for optimal blood glucose results with exercise. Taking the following steps can help you fine-tune your diabetes management plan as you increase exercise in your lifestyle:

1. Gather information.

▶ Monitor your blood glucose and keep a record of your readings.
▶ Note things that may affect your blood glucose levels, including
  ▶ diabetes medications that you take, their dosages, and when you take them in relation to the time of day that you do an activity;
  ▶ the timing of activity sessions in relation to when you eat meals and snacks;
  ▶ what foods you eat for meals and snacks;
  ▶ stress or any other factor that may influence blood glucose levels on a given day and how they change with activity.

2. Study the information that you collect.

▶ See if you can find repeating patterns or trends in how your blood glucose levels change with activity.

▶ Look for reasons that explain how blood glucose changes when you are active.

3. Use the information you collect to take action.

▶ Consider if your diabetes management plan may need to be adjusted and discuss this with your diabetes care provider; helpful adjustments may include:

   ▶ changing the time of day that you do physical activity;

   ▶ increasing or decreasing how much activity you do, for example adjusting the intensity or duration of an exercise session;

   ▶ changing the timing of your meals or snacks in relation to your activity sessions;

   ▶ modifying the amounts or types of foods that you eat before, during, or after doing activity;

   ▶ changing timing or dosages of medication(s).

4. Try out your modified management strategies.

5. See how the changes you tried worked.

▶ If they worked, great! If not, try the above steps again until you find what works best when it comes to reaching your glucose goals.

Record keeping

Record keeping is important when you are striving to understand how changes in your diabetes management plan affect your blood glucose levels. Figure 5-2 provides an outline for collecting key information that will help you see what happens to your blood glucose level when you exercise and how to reach your glucose goals with activity. To illustrate this, let's look at how Mike, a 52-year-old man who has had type 2 diabetes for 3 years, used this record to get a handle on his blood glucose level and improve his glucose control by doing more physical activity.

Getting on track—Mike's records

Mike monitored his blood glucose two or three times every day; in the morning before breakfast and in the evening before and/or after dinner. He took his diabetes medications, and tried to follow a meal plan. However, he did not keep records. He recently had an appointment with his doctor and found that his A1C was 7.8 percent (higher than his goal). He had also gained a few pounds. Mike and his physician discussed the benefits of gradually increasing daily physical activity, and Mike decided he would like to work up to doing at least 45 minutes of daily activity. He wanted to see if this would improve his blood glucose control, help with his efforts to lose some weight, and improve his heart health. He and his doctor also talked about increasing his blood glucose monitoring for a few weeks to four times per day and keeping a record so that Mike, with the support of diabetes educators, could find ways to include more activity in his management plan and improve his blood glucose control.

Mike used the *Daily Diabetes Self-Management Record* (Figure 5-2) to gather information about his diabetes management. In his record, he noted:

- ▶ his blood glucose goals;
- ▶ the diabetes medications that he took, including dosages and times;
- ▶ his blood glucose readings from his meter;
- ▶ variances in his food intake;
- ▶ the types of activities that he did, the time of day, the amount of time of each activity session, and the perceived effort;
- ▶ factors that may have explained blood glucose readings.

Mike then looked at the information he collected. He drew a square around every blood glucose reading that was above his goal range and a circle around readings that were below his goal range. Mike identified some patterns:

- ▶ His blood glucose tended to be high in the mornings, both before breakfast and two hours after his meal. When he did some physical activity in the morning, his glucose levels improved.
- ▶ Two hours after lunch, his blood glucose tended to be in his goal range.

Figure 5-2. Daily Diabetes Self-Management Record

	Breakfast					Lunch					Dinner					Physical Activity/ Other
	BG Time:	Meds	Breakfast Time: Carbs:	BG Time:	BG Time:	Meds	Lunch Time: Carbs:	BG Time:	BG Time:	Meds	Dinner Time: Carbs:	BG Time:				Type, time of day, how long, effort
Sun																Other variables:
Mon																Other variables:
Tue																Other variables:
Wed																Other variables:
Thur																Other variables:
Fri																Other variables:
Sat																Other variables:

Key Instructions for Figure 5-2

Diabetes Medications: Note what diabetes medications you take, dosages, and time(s) that you take them.

Blood Glucose Goals: Write down your schedule for blood glucose monitoring and your goals at each time.

Day: Under the day of the week, note the date.

Activity Record: Note each session of activity that you do.

> Type: Note the form of activity that you do—for example, walking, stretching, or yard work.
>
> Time: Note the time of day that you do an activity and the duration of each session—for example, 8:30–9:00 AM walked for 30 min.
>
> Effort: Use perceived exertion (see chapter 3, Figure 3-1) to identify how hard or difficult the activity seemed while you were doing it.

Blood Glucose Record: Note blood glucose values before and/or 2 hours after your meal(s). Talk to your doctor or health care team about monitoring and the best schedule for you to follow, especially if you are unsure when you should test. Draw a *circle* around any BG that is *below* and a *square* around any BG that is *above* your goal range.

Other: Note any factors or variances, like stress, time of day that you do an activity, illness, or food, that may influence your blood glucose readings. Note results of any additional blood glucose tests that you do, for example, before and after activity.

Food Notes: Note the time(s) of your meals and snacks—especially in relation to exercise times and any variances from your usual way of eating (for example, eating more or less than usual, eating later or earlier than usual, or eating foods that are "unusual" for you).

Note: Most blood glucose meters now have data management systems, and some meters even enable you to input information about physical activity, food, and medications. With some you can even download results to your computer or a Web site and create complete reports. if you prefer to go "high tech," talk with your health care provider or diabetes educator about data management systems and specific diabetes apps for your smartphone that might be helpful to you.

> ▶ His evening blood glucose—which he measured on alternate days, either 2 hours after his meal or at bedtime—was too high. Doing some evening activity helped this come closer to his target. Stress and overeating may have been contributing factors. He found that staying with his eating plan was most challenging at dinnertime and in the evening.

He used the information to take action.

Based on the information that he collected and the blood glucose patterns that he identified, Mike decided to try the following strategies to improve his glucose control:

- Get up early and do 20 minutes of fitness walking or go to his neighborhood pool to swim laps in the morning.
- Do at least 30 minutes of activity in the evening (either walking, yard work, or weight lifting).
- Re-focus on his eating patterns and portion sizes, especially in the evening; get out and do some physical activity or get busy with something else to prevent unnecessary snacking.

He evaluated the effectiveness of these new management strategies.

Mike continued to keep records, and when he studied them, he found that his blood glucose control improved when he was consistent about his physical activity routine—exercising at least every other day for 30–45 minutes. He found that with his new focus on fitness, he started making healthier food choices, too. He discovered that keeping records increased his self-awareness and was actually very motivational! The follow-up appointment with his diabetes educator was also beneficial because he was able to share his records, and the very useful information in them. Mike and his educator were able to make a few adjustments in his routine, which further improved his glucose control.

The guidelines and strategies that Mike used can help you achieve and maintain optimal blood glucose control with activity. These guidelines are general and the strategies Mike used are simply suggestions of techniques to try. Both are meant to provide you with a foundation and a starting point. However, you have your own history with diabetes and your own exercise goals. How you decide to fit physical activity into your daily routine is unique to you. The skills you learned in this chapter can help you develop and fine-tune your methods of doing this for long-term success while achieving the best possible glucose control and overall health.

Become more aware through activity

One of the great things about physical activity is that it is a healthy habit, and it tends to help us focus on other lifestyle habits that also can improve our health and well-being. When we do physical activity, we are clued in to how we feel—great, energetic, sluggish, tired—and this helps us to evaluate why we feel a given way. Many athletes—runners, for

Figure 5-3. Mike's Daily Diabetes Self-Management Record

	Breakfast					Lunch				Dinner			Physical Activity/Other
	BG Time: 7:30	Meds	Breakfast Time: 7:45 Carbs: 60 g	BG Time: 10:30	BG Time: 12:30	Meds	Lunch Time: 12:45 Carbs: 60 g	BG Time: 3:00	BG Time: 6:30	Meds	Dinner Time: 7:00 Carbs: 75 g	BG Time: 9:30	Type, time of day, how long, effort
Sun	152	Glipizide 10 mg. Metformin 500 mg.	Cereal 1 c. Milk 1 c. Banana 1 lg Toast 1 sl	175	98		Sandwich 2 Bread Lg apple	133	128	Glipizide 5 mg. Metformin 500 mg.	4 oz Steak Lg Potato Salad 2 bites Cake	201	Walk 20 min. at noon Light/Easy Other: ate dinner out, larger portions than usual and dessert
Mon	146	Glipizide 10 mg. Metformin 500 mg.	Bagel 3 oz Lt Cream Cheese 2 T Orange	139	116		Sandwich 2 Bread Lg Pear	149	108	Glipizide 5 mg. Metformin 500 mg.	Spaghetti 1.5 c. Salad Roll	188	Water exercise 7:30 - 8:30 AM; Moderate: RPE = 12
Tues	143	Glipizide 10 mg. Metformin 500 mg.	Cereal 1 c. Milk 1 c. Banana 1 lg Toast 1 sl		91		Pizza 1/2 sl (Sausage & Mushroom) Salad with no-fat dressing SF soda	69 .5 c OJ (15 g.)	156	Glipizide 5 mg. Metformin 500 mg.	4 oz Chicken Rice 3/4 c Vegs. 1 c Roll 12 Grapes	107	Walk for 45 min. 6:30 - 7:15 AM Moderate: RPE = 12 Walk for 20 min. lunch. Work in yard 50 min. evening Other: smaller than usual lunch, not enough carbs? More activity than usual
Wed													
Thu													
Fri													
Sat													

example—keep daily logs of how they feel during workouts and take note of the things that occurred that may have affected their performance. They use this information to fine-tune their training methods and create a competitive edge.

Being physically active when you have diabetes takes some effort, especially at first. But like the athlete, logging your diabetes management and physical activity can be very helpful. Blood glucose monitoring, record keeping, and learning to identify blood glucose patterns are skills that will help you fine-tune strategies for successfully increasing physical activity in your daily routine. As you go about this process, you will find yourself becoming more aware of the interactions among the foods you eat, the medications that you take, stress levels, and other factors that affect how you feel and how your blood glucose changes when you are physically active. The benefit of having this level of awareness is that it can help you to make other positive lifestyle changes in addition to being physically active. You will find yourself, in many ways, noticing your lifestyle choices and being surprisingly persistent about your diabetes self-management and overall health.

By committing to becoming more physically active you begin to take charge and successfully self-manage your diabetes for optimal glucose control, improved health, and a heightened sense of well-being.

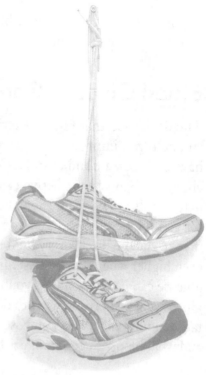

Chapter 6

KEEP YOUR BLOOD GLUCOSE IN BALANCE WITH PHYSICAL ACTIVITY

By now you've seen that physical activity is not only good, it's great for those with pre-diabetes or diabetes. Being physically active helps you manage your condition by

- ▶ lowering blood glucose;
- ▶ improving the body's ability to use insulin;
- ▶ improving cardiovascular risk factors;
- ▶ reducing high blood pressure;
- ▶ raising your HDL, or "good," cholesterol level;
- ▶ reducing high triglyceride levels;
- ▶ helping you lose weight or maintain a healthier weight.

In order to achieve these health benefits, however, you must know how to make self-management decisions when you exercise. Most importantly, monitoring your blood glucose levels with exercise helps you to measure your success.

Blood Glucose Control with Activity

The likelihood that physical activity will lower your blood glucose level and help you improve your glucose control is real. However, when you have diabetes, a number of factors can affect how your blood glucose changes when you are active (Table 6-1), and the changes you experience may not always be predictable. For example, in some instances, it is possible for your blood glucose to fall too low when you exercise. Yet, in other cases, if your glucose level is very high to begin with, it can stay elevated or rise even higher when you exercise. In either situation, managing your blood glucose can be tricky unless you understand why you are experiencing blood glucose challenges and what to do about them So, as a first step, it is important to know what blood glucose level is considered high, what level is low, and what blood glucose range is best when you exercise.

Physical activity and high blood glucose levels

It is best to have acceptable blood glucose control before you begin a new activity program, especially if it includes more vigorous exercise than you are used to. If your blood glucose levels are always out of range—and especially if they have been out of range for a while—see your health care provider before you begin doing more activity. Your diabetes medications or eating plan may need some adjustments to help bring your glucose level toward a healthier and safer range. Always think about possible other causes of high blood glucose levels, such as an infection, a cold, or the flu. If your glucose level is high (hyperglycemia), you'll have to decide whether or not to exercise. When making this decision, consider the following guidelines:

▶ If your blood glucose is moderately high due to issues such as emotional stress or eating too much at a meal, physical activity will usually have a positive blood glucose–lowering effect.

▶ When your blood glucose is high due to illness or infection, use common sense. It is best to wait until you feel well. Check with your health care provider if you have questions or concerns about your readiness to resume activity.

▶ If your blood glucose is 300 mg/dl or greater, use caution and consider what could be contributing to your high glucose level. Depending on your assessment, it may be OK to exercise or it may be better to delay doing activity until your glucose level is better controlled.

   ▷ If you have any concerns, check with your health care provider before resuming exercise.

   ▷ If your blood glucose is too high, you may even benefit from doing some light to moderate activity, especially if your glucose is elevated after a meal. However, use caution, and be certain to drink plenty of water before, during, and after any activity you do.

▶ If you think your blood glucose is elevated due to a reason such as illness or infection, wait to exercise.

▶ High blood glucose levels can cause you to feel tired and fatigued, especially when you attempt physical activity. That is because your muscles aren't supplied with the extra glucose and energy that they need for exercise. As a result, doing activity can feel more difficult than usual.

▶ When your blood glucose is high, it is easy to become dehydrated because you lose body fluid through frequent urination. Doing exercise when you are dehydrated can be stressful on your heart and cardiovascular system and contribute to poor body temperature regulation and overheating. So, make an extra effort to drink plenty of water or other non-caloric fluids if you exercise when your glucose level is high.

Though physical activity alone will not necessarily correct very high blood glucose levels, it does contribute to better overall health and to improved long-term blood glucose control, especially when it is part of a complete diabetes management plan. Healthy eating, blood glucose monitoring, and working with your health care provider and diabetes educator to assure that diabetes medications are appropriately adjusted are also essential.

People with type 1 diabetes are more likely to experience high blood ketone levels than people with type 2, but ketones can appear in anyone with diabetes. The combination of very high blood glucose levels and ketones indicate that you don't have enough circulating insulin to meet your body's needs. And anytime you don't have enough insulin, your muscles can't get the glucose they need to meet their demand for extra energy during physical activity. When your muscles sense that they don't have enough glucose, your liver responds by increasing glucose production. In addition, your body rapidly breaks down its fat stores for energy; ketones are by-products of this breakdown. If ketones form faster than your body can get rid of them in urine, they build up in the blood, and it becomes too acidic. As a result, blood glucose and ketone levels can continue to rise and you can become dehydrated and at risk for a condition called diabetic ketoacidosis (DKA). If not promptly and adequately treated, DKA can lead to coma, shock, and even death. So, although physical activity usually helps to lower blood glucose levels, this may not be the case if your blood glucose is very high. This can be an important reason to see your health care provider and achieve better control before resuming exercise.

Physical activity and low blood glucose levels

In some situations, blood glucose levels can fall too low. This is called hypoglycemia. However, not everyone is at risk for hypoglycemia, which is considered a glucose reading of 70 mg/dl or less on your meter and/or the presence of symptoms (Table 6-1).

If you have pre-diabetes you do not run any greater risk of experiencing hypoglycemia with activity than someone who doesn't have pre-diabetes. When you have type 2 diabetes, the possibility that you will develop hypoglycemia with exercise is higher *only* if you take insulin injections or certain types of oral diabetes medications that can increase risk of hypoglycemia (Table 6-2). Typically, consistent physical activity will lead to a gradual and beneficial lowering of your blood glucose level and will help you maintain your glucose in a desirable range. So use this to your advantage!

A key point to remember for those with pre-diabetes or type 2 diabetes: Because you are not likely to experience activity-related hypoglycemia, you usually don't need to eat extra food when you do physical activity. Extra food can prevent you from benefiting from the blood glucose–lowering effect that results from doing activity, and it can contribute to lack of progress with weightloss efforts.

Table 6-1. Factors that Influence the Effect of Activity on Blood Glucose Levels

▶ Overall diabetes control

▶ Blood glucose level before exercise, which is influenced by:
  ▷ Diabetes medications
  ▷ Time of day of exercise
  ▷ Time of exercise in relation to last meal or snack
  ▷ Emotions such as stress or feelings of anxiety
  ▷ Level of fitness
  ▷ Length of activity session
  ▷ Intensity of activity

A key point to remember if you are at risk for hypoglycemia: If you are trying to lose weight, routinely eating extra food and carbohydrate when exercising can limit your success with weight loss and can prevent long-term improvements in blood glucose control as you increase activity. However, when you exercise, you should always be prepared to treat low blood glucose with a source of carbohydrate that will rapidly raise your glucose level if it falls too low. If you suspect that your blood glucose is low, test to verify first before treating with carbohydrate. It is best to monitor your blood glucose before and after exercise if you experience unexpected glucose variations. If you find you often have to eat extra carbohydrate to treat hypoglycemia, consider these other options:

▶ Talk to your health care provider to make sure the dosages of your medications and the times that you take them are correct. It is possible that, as you lose a few pounds and become more fit, your medication dosages will need to be reduced.

▶ Consider changing the time of day you exercise in relation to your usual meal and snack times. For example, plan an activity session 1–2 hours after a meal instead of after a long period of time without food.

If you have type 2 diabetes and you take one of the medications that puts you at a higher risk of experiencing hypoglycemia, you should be aware of the signs and symptoms of hypoglycemia (Table 6-3), how to treat hypoglycemia with a carbohydrate (CHO) source that will quickly raise your glucose level (Figure 6-1), and what actions to take to prevent hypoglycemia from happening again (Table 6-4).

If you are on insulin therapy, there is a possibility that your blood glucose level could fall too low with exercise. So, be aware of symptoms of hypoglycemia (Table 6-3), the steps to take to treat lows (Figure 6-1), which carbohydrate (CHO) sources are best for rapidly raising your glucose level (Table 6-4), and steps to take to prevent exercise-related hypoglycemia from happening again.

Table 6-2. Oral and Injectable Diabetes Medications and Hypoglycemia Risk with Activity

ORAL MEDICATIONS THAT DO INCREASE RISK OF HYPOGLYCEMIA

Sulfonylureas
Glyburide (DiaBeta®, Micronase®, Glynase Prestabs®)
Glipizide (Glucotrol®/Glucotrol XL®)
Glimepiride (Amaryl®)
Meglitinide
Repaglinide (Prandin®)
Nateglinide (Starlix®)

Combinations
Glyburide plus metformin (Glucovance®)
Glipizide plus metformin (Metaglip®)

ORAL MEDICATIONS THAT DON'T INCREASE RISK OF HYPOGLYCEMIA

Alpha-glucosidase inhibitors[a,b]
Acarbose (Precose®)
Miglitol (Glycet®)

Biguanides[c]
Metformin (Glucophage®)

Thiazolidinediones[a,c]
Rosiglitazone (Avandia®)
Pioglitazone (Actos®)

Combinations
Rosiglitazone plus metformin (Avandamet®)

GLP-1 Receptor Agonists
Exenatide (Byetta™)[a]
Exenatide Extended Release (Bydureon™)[a]
Liraglutide (Victoza®)

Amylin Analog
Pramlintide acetate (Symlin®)[a]

DPP-4 Inhibitors
Saxagliptin (Onglyza™)[a]
Sitagliptin (Januvia®)[a]
Linagliptin (Tradjenta™)[a]

[a] Can contribute to hypoglycemia when used as combination therapy with insulin or sulfonylureas.
[b] Glucose must be used as treatment for hypoglycemia; alpha-glucosidase inhibitors prevent sucrose (table sugar) from being an effective treatment.
[c] Hypoglycemia is possible with long-duration exercise.

A key point to remember if you take insulin: Blood glucose monitoring before and after exercise sessions will help you learn how your blood glucose changes with activity. It will also help you make good decisions about when to exercise based on your blood glucose readings. Remember to test any time you suspect your blood glucose is low so that you can take steps to treat hypoglycemia quickly and correctly. If you take insulin, a SFU (sulfonylurea), SFU combination, or meglitinide it is possible to develop exercise-related hypoglycemia during or several hours (up to 36 hours) after the activity has ended.

Table 6-3. Signs and Symptoms of Hypoglycemia

► Blood glucose reading of 70 mg/dl or less on your meter*

► Sweating/changes in body temperature†

► Trembling

► Tingling

► Difficulty concentrating/ thinking slowly

► Lightheadedness/dizziness

► Slurred speech

► Blurred vision

► Lack of coordination

► Tiredness, fatigue, sleepiness

► Pounding heart/fast pulse†

► Heavy or rapid breathing†

► Hunger

► General feeling that "something's not right"

* A blood glucose value of 70 mg/dl or less indicates hypoglycemia; always test when you notice symptoms.
† Note these symptoms of hypoglycemia may be "masked" with physical activity because they also result from doing exercise.

Activity, insulin, and hypoglycemia: Additional considerations

► Always be prepared with carbohydrate sources to treat hypoglycemia. If you do vigorous or prolonged exercise—lasting more than about 45 minutes—you may need to take in extra carbohydrate to keep your blood glucose level in a safe range. An intake of 15–30 grams of carbohydrate every 15–30 minutes of activity is usually enough to keep blood glucose levels from falling too low. Blood glucose monitoring can help you make good decisions about whether or not you need to eat additional carbohydrate. Remember that overeating can prevent improvements in blood glucose levels and can contribute unnecessary extra calories.

► Know when the insulin you take is peaking, or most actively lowering your blood glucose (Table 6-5). Exercise increases blood flow, which may increase how fast your insulin goes to work. If you exercise when insulin is peaking, you are more likely to experience a large drop in your glucose level than if you exercise before or after your insulin is most active.

▶ If you often have low blood glucose levels with exercise or you find that you need to consume a lot of extra carbohydrate to keep your glucose level in a safe range, your insulin dosage(s) may need to be adjusted. Talk to your health care provider about this.

Figure 6-1. How to Handle Hypoglycemia with Activity

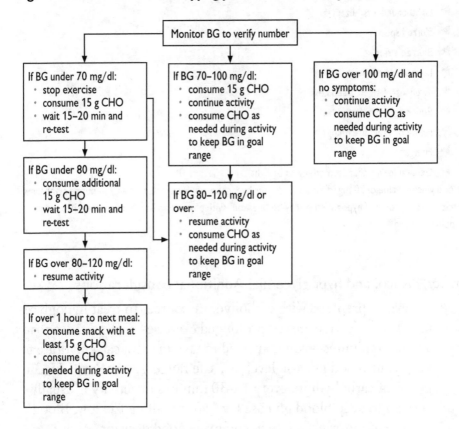

Key: BG = blood glucose; CHO = carbohydrate; g = grams

©2006, The American Dietetic Association. *Sports Nutrition: A Guide for the Professional Working with Active People.* Adapted with permission.

Table 6-4. Carbohydrate (CHO) Sources for Treating Hypoglycemia with Activity

CHO SOURCE	AMOUNT	CHO GRAMS SUPPLIED	CALORIES*
Glucose Tablets	3	15 g	60
Insta Glucos™	18 g	15 g	60
Glutose™	40 g	15 g	64
Fruit Juice	1/2 cup	15–20 g	60–80
Fruit Sauce	1 pouch (90 g)	15 g	60
Gatorade®	1 cup	12 g	50
Soft Drinks (Regular)	1/2–2/3 cup	15 g	55–60
Lifesavers®	8	15 g	60
Gum Drops	6	15 g	65
Fruit Roll-Up®	1	12 g	50
Raisins	2 Tbsp	17 g	75
NutraGrain Bar®	1/2	15 g	70
Power Bar®	1/3	15 g	60

NOTE: All sources of carbohydrate have calories. Be aware of portion sizes! Overtreating hypoglycemia may cause blood glucose levels to be too high later on and can prevent long-term weightloss success.

Table 6-5. Insulin Time/Action Profiles

TYPE OF INSULIN	ONSET	PEAK	DURATION
Rapid-Acting			
Lispro (Humalog)	<15 min	0.5–2.5 hr	3–4 hr
Aspart (Novolog)	<15 min	1–3 hr	3–5 hr
Glulisine (Apidra)	<15 min	1–3 hr	3–5 hr
Short-Acting			
Regular	0.5–1 hr	2–3 hr	6–8 hr
Intermediate-Acting			
NPH	2–4 hr	4–10 hr	10–16 hr
Long-Acting			
Glargine (Lantus)	1–2 hr	Peakless	24 hr
Detemir (Levemir)	2 hr	4–8 hr (dose dependent)	up to 24 hr

Other Exercise Safety Considerations

Every physical activity session should be a safe and enjoyable experience! That said, there are a few exercise safety considerations that everyone with pre-diabetes or diabetes should know. These are especially important for anyone who has diabetes complications.

Making safe activity choices, especially if you have complications or physical limitations, is a first step toward exercise safety. *Table 1-1. Exercising Safely with Diabetes Complications* (page 9) identifies activities that are safe for you and those that require caution when you have complications. Always talk to your doctor if you are not sure if an activity is a good option for you to do.

Beyond choosing beneficial and safe activities, there are additional safety tips that you should follow whenever you are active. Although most of these points require a little attention and preplanning, they don't take a lot of time or effort. However, they contribute in a big way to exercise safety. Some of these are sensible for anyone who exercises; others are specific to individuals with diabetes.

General safety points

▶ Always warm up your muscles at the beginning of an activity session and cool down at the end. Remember, your heart is a muscle and requires a warm-up and cool-down too!

▶ Keep exercise intensity (or effort) at a moderate and comfortable level

▶ Avoid doing activity in extremely hot or cold temperatures—choose indoor options when the weather is extreme

▶ Drink at least 2 cups of fluid within 2 hours of starting exercise and drink fluids often during exercise (try to drink 1/2 to 1 cup of fluid every 15 minutes)

▶ Wear good-quality footwear that is appropriate for the activity you plan to do. Shoes with silica gel or air mid-soles are a good choice for weight-bearing activities like walking because they are built to reduce stress on the feet and joints

▶ Wear clothing that is appropriate for the exercise climate (warm in the winter, cool in the summer)

- ▶ Stop doing an activity if you feel any pain, discomfort, shortness of breath, or light-headedness; report unusual symptoms to your health care provider

Diabetes-specific safety points

- ▶ Always wear diabetes identification
- ▶ Always have your meter and carry a treatment for hypoglycemia
- ▶ If you take insulin or an oral medication that increases hypoglycemia risk, monitor your glucose before and after you exercise
- ▶ Inform someone that you have diabetes and tell him or her what to do to help you if your blood glucose drops too low during an activity session
- ▶ Carefully inspect your feet for blisters, redness, or other signs of irritation both before and after doing activity
- ▶ Wear clean socks (made with a material that reduces friction and pulls moisture away from your feet like CoolMax®, MicroSafe®, polypropylene, or acrylic) that fit smoothly into your shoe.

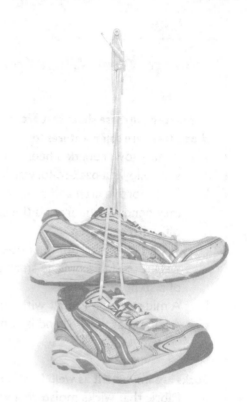

Chapter 7
WALK YOUR WAY TO HEALTH

"One step, another step, one step, and another...." Recall the words of the wise tortoise as he won the race with the hare. He won by walking along steadily, always moving toward his goal of winning. The similarities to making progress with fitness goals are pretty striking. Those who try to do too much too fast (and have unrealistic expectations) are less likely to succeed, if not in the short term then in the long. Those who realize that becoming more fit and healthy takes time and commitment—a whole lifetime, in fact—are more likely to be successful at reaching goals.

Walking is simple, can be enjoyable, and is something most everyone can do—including you! It is great for improving health and overall fitness. Walking has very few disadvantages but many advantages. For example, walking

▶ is inexpensive;
▶ does not require special skill or equipment (see the box, *What to Wear When You Walk*);

What to Wear When You Walk

Shoes

It is best to purchase shoes that are specifically made for walking. When buying shoes, there are some features to consider:

▶ A fairly low, rounded heel and an upward bend at the toe so the shoe allows a back-to-forward rolling foot motion from heel to toe

▶ A supportive arch and a flex point that bends where your foot naturally bends—right around the ball of the foot—just before you "toe off" with each step

▶ Slight flexibility from the outer to inner toe box to allow your weight to shift from the small to big toe as you "toe off" at the end of a step

▶ A mid-sole that is built with materials that reduce stress on the foot

▶ A shoe that fits well and is comfortable

Socks

Socks are important as well. Look for these features in a sock:

▶ Fabric that wicks moisture away from your foot, such as CoolMax®, MicroSafe®, Dri-Fit®, or Sorbtek® (stay away from cotton)

▶ A smooth fit that does not bunch or bind

▶ Padding where it is needed—at the ball of the foot, instep, and heel

▶ A double layer, which may help reduce friction and blistering for some people

Clothing

Choose clothing that is right for the climate.

▶ In hot weather:
  ▷ Wear lightweight, light-colored clothing
  ▷ Look for fabrics like CoolMax® or polypropylene that transport moisture away from your skin

▶ In cool weather, wear layers (add as many as you need depending on the climate):
  ▷ For the inner layer (next to your skin), wear a moisture-wicking fabric to keep your skin comfortable and dry
  ▷ For the middle layer, add a fleece or wool sweater for warmth
  ▷ For the outer layer, wear a jacket made from a fabric that will protect from wind, cold, or rain, such as nylon or Gore-Tex

- can fit easily into any schedule and be done in short amounts of time;
- is a natural movement that is easy to do correctly and hard to do wrong;
- is safe and carries little risk of injury;
- is pleasant and relaxing;
- promotes social interaction and friendships;
- and is easy to stick with.

Considering all of these great advantages of walking, why not get started?

The First Step

When beginning a walking program, your first step is to gather information about how much walking you do as you go about a usual day. For the first week, don't alter your typical amount of activity. Keep a tally of the number of minutes you spend walking or use a pedometer (see the box *Tips for Finding and Using a Pedometer*) to count the number of steps you take each day. A pedometer doesn't have to be expensive, and once you start counting your steps with one, you'll find you have a nifty gadget that is great for figuring out your step-count numbers, setting goals, keeping track of progress, and staying motivated to reach your goals.

The first week of your walking program is a good time to get in the habit of keeping a walking log (Figure 7-1). Write down the amount of time you spend walking and/or the number of steps you take throughout the day. Note whether this amount of walking is more, less, or a usual amount for you. Finally, note how much effort you feel you exerted for the amount of walking you did (see the *Borg Rating of Perceived Exertion*

Figure 7-1. Sample Walking Log

Week _____

	Mon.	Tues.	Wed.	Thurs.	Fri.	Sat.	Sun.
Minutes of Walking							
Number of Steps							
Perception (RPE)							

Tips for Finding and Using a Pedometer

Where to Find a Pedometer

▶ Most athletic stores have pedometers, but you can also order them online or through other mail-order options.

▶ A basic pedometer model records step counts only, and this is all you really need to know. However, higher-priced models may also estimate and record the distance you walk and the number of calories you burn. Some models hold downloadable data and even connect to a Web site to chart your progress and graph your daily activity.

▶ It is a good idea to purchase a safety strap for your pedometer to prevent it from falling off and being damaged or lost.

▶ Pedometer resources:

▷ Accusplit: www.accusplit.com 800-935-1996

▷ American Diabetes Association: www.diabetes.org 800-232-6733

▷ New Lifestyles: www.new-lifestyles.com 816-373-9969

▷ fitbit : www.fitbit.com

▷ Omron: www.omronwebstore.com 866-896-5452

[**NOTE:** If you have a smartphone, consider downloading and trying out a pedometer app to help keep track of your daily step count.]

How to Use a Pedometer

▶ A pedometer should be fastened to a belt or waistband directly above the midpoint of the front of your thigh. (Pedometers measure step counts by recording vertical hip movement, so position is important.)

▶ It should be secured so that it stays in a vertical and upright position. If it slips, it may not count the steps you take.

▶ The cover on the pedometer must be closed or it may not accurately register steps.

▶ At the beginning of each day, reset your pedometer to "0" to clear the previous day's count. Then, do a quick accuracy check by walking a set number of steps (for example, 30). Keep track of the number of steps yourself and check that your pedometer has recorded the correct number. For the rest of the day, let your pedometer do the counting for you.

▶ Most pedometers have the best accuracy when you walk at a 2- to 4-mile-per-hour pace. If you walk very slowly or if you run, some steps may not be recorded.

Scale on page 34). By the end of the first week, you will have gathered useful information that will help you get started.

Now that you have this information to work with, you can figure out your "baseline" minutes of walking or steps per day. To do this:

1. Add up the number of minutes you walked or the number of steps you took for each of the seven days of the week (Mon.+ Tues.+ Wed., etc.) to get a total for the week.
2. Divide the total number(s) by 7 to get an average number of minutes or steps per day. The average is your "baseline" number, which gives you a starting point to build on as you begin your walking routine.

The Second Step

The second step of a walking program is to build more steps into your day. As you do this, remember: "slow and steady wins the race." Doing too much too fast can lead to burnout and setbacks. Be patient, make steady progress, and keep going.

Setting walking goals

Goal setting can help you make gradual, steady, and successful progress toward building more steps into your day. Here are some strategies for setting goals for walking:

1. First, look at your baseline amount of walking (either in minutes per day or steps per day) and then check Table 7-1 to see what activity level this amount falls under (low, low-active, somewhat active, or active).
2. Next think about why you want to begin a walking program. Do you want to lose or maintain your current weight, lower your blood glucose level, lower your blood pressure, or reduce stress? Or, do you simply want to feel better and have more stamina?
3. Look at Table 7-1 and note how much walking you'll need to do each day to get the benefits you desire. For example, if you want "better health," work up to at least 7,500 steps per day.
4. Build onto your "baseline" by setting a SMART goal (see Chapter 2) to help you reach the level of walking that is associated with the health, fitness, and lifestyle benefits you want to achieve.

Table 7-1. Level of Activity by Step Counts and Minutes Walking

Level of Activity	Step Count/Minutes of Walking Per Day	Step-Count Goals and Related Benefits
Low	<5000 steps/45–50 min.	Amount of walking in a "normal day"
Low–Active	5,000–7,499 steps/50–75 min.	Gradually improve level of fitness
Somewhat Active	7,500–9,999 steps/75–100 min.	Improve health and reduce risk of chronic disease
Active	10,000–>15,000 steps/100–150 min.	Prevent weight gain or regain after weight loss*

Requires structured time dedicated to walking (outside on a track, on a treadmill, etc.) in addition to an effort to take more steps throughout the day

What's your pace?

Table 7-2 is a sample 12-week fitness walking program that can help guide you toward a more active lifestyle. However, the rate at which you decide to increase your amount of walking may be a bit faster or a bit more gradual than this. As you add steps to your routine, keep these numbers in mind:

▶ 100 steps takes about 1 minute of walking.
▶ 500 steps is about 1/4 mile and takes about 5 minutes of walking.
▶ 1,000 steps is about 1/2 mile and takes about 10 minutes of walking.
▶ 2,000 steps is about 1 mile and takes about 20 minutes of walking.
▶ 5,000 steps is about 2 1/2 miles and takes about 45 minutes of walking.
▶ 10,000 steps is about 5 miles and takes 90–100 minutes of walking.

Table 7-2. Sample 12-Week Fitness Walking Program

Week	Slow		Brisk		Slow		Total	
	Min.	Steps	Min.	Steps	Min.	Steps	Min.	Steps
1	Keep track of your usual amount of daily walking to determine your baseline numbers in minutes of walking or steps per day.							
2	5	500	5–8	500–800	5	500	15–18	1500–1800
3	5	500	8–11	800–1100	5	500	18–21	1800–2100
4	5	500	11–14	1100–1400	5	500	21–24	2100–2400
5	5	500	14–17	1400–1700	5	500	24–27	2400–2700
6	5	500	17-20	1700–2000	5	500	27–30	2700–3000
7	5	500	20–25	2000–2500	5	500	30–35	3000–3500
8	5	500	25–30	2500–3000	5	500	35–40	3500–4000
9	5	500	30–35	3000–3500	5	500	40–45	4000–4500
10	5	500	35–45	3500–4500	5	500	45–55	4500–5500
11	5	500	45–55	4500–5500	5	500	55–65	5500–6500
12 (and on)	5	500	Maintain or continue to increase by 5 min. per week until you reach your goals		5	500	Maintain or continue to increase	

Always begin with slow, warm-up walking and stretching and end with slow, cool-down walking and stretching.

You can get health benefits by walking at any speed. But if you're looking for greater fitness gains—weight loss, stronger muscles, increased heart/lung stamina—experts have a few tips. As always, check with your health care provider before stepping up your fitness program.

- Make it brisk. A leisurely stroll will help relax and energize you, but a brisk walk (3–4 miles per hour) will give your heart a good workout and burn more calories. Aim to boost aerobic fitness by walking at least 1.5 miles (about 3,000 steps) per day at a brisk pace. Just be sure to walk at a pace that allows you to pass the "talk test."
- Take more steps. If you want to speed up your walk, don't lengthen your stride. That can feel awkward and also cause pain in your knees, shins, and feet. Instead, step more quickly, all the while maintaining a comfortable, natural stride.
- Push off with your toes. If you push off with your toes at the end of each step, this will add power to your walk. As you push off, imagine that you are going to show someone who is walking behind you the sole of your shoe.
- Pump your arms. Swinging your arms down by your sides as you walk can cause discomfort in the back. Instead, bend your elbows, hold them close to your body at waist level, and pump them back and forth as you walk. This will help you go faster and will prevent stress on your lower back.
- Focus on posture and form. Pull your shoulders up, your stomach muscles in, and stand tall when you walk. Avoid swaying excessively from side to side. Lean slightly forward at the waist, keep your chin up, and look forward toward a distant point.

Remember, the amount of walking that you decide to do is up to you. If you get great results by adding 30 minutes of walking to your daily routine, this may be enough for you. However, if you find that 30 minutes is not enough to get the results you want or if you enjoy walking so much that you want to do more, decide on another amount that is right for you. The most important thing is to find a routine that works for you and that you enjoy. Then it will be easy for you to stick with it!

The Third Step

During the first months of building your walking program, it is important to get into the habit of walking more throughout the day, including taking a planned, structured walk. Though the amount of walking you decide to do will depend on your goals, consistency is always important. Remember to use the strategies covered in chapter 2. They are proven to support success. Also remember that it takes about 6 months to create a firm physical activity habit. The positive results you see—having more energy, stamina, and endurance, seeing muscles tone up, and developing a newfound confidence—can be very reinforcing and will help you stick with it.

The third, and final, step of your walking program is to develop strategies that will help you continue to stick with it long-term. Maintaining any physical activity routine can, at times, be challenging due to things that "get in the way," like schedule changes, hectic or busy times, waning motivation, or boredom with an exercise routine. However, consistency remains important. So, here are some ideas for staying with your program:

▶ Keep a record. This will help keep your attention focused on your walking routine and help you face backsliding early, before it becomes a more serious relapse.

▶ Continue to set goals and to reward yourself. For example, set your sights on walking in a community walk that will raise funds for a cause that you care about. Sometimes just the t-shirt at the end of the walk can make the whole thing worthwhile.

▶ Keep it interesting. Find three or four walking routes that you enjoy.

▶ Have both indoor and outdoor options for walking.

▶ Keep it social. Walk with a neighbor, friend, or coworker, or even form a walking group.

▶ Mix it up and vary your walking routine. On some days, walk longer distances but slow down the pace a bit, on other days pick up the pace but shorten the distance, or do intervals and alternate slow and fast walking paces on another day.

▶ Look at the positives. Make a list of all the benefits you are getting from walking.

Finally, think about all the effort you have put into building your walking program and getting into shape and consider how much more you can do now than you maybe ever thought you could. If you stay focused on all the positives, it will be hard to go back to a less active lifestyle.

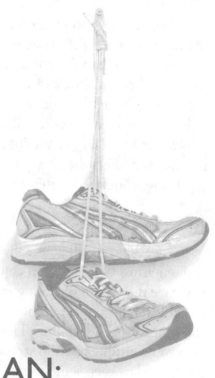

Chapter 8

AN ACTIVITY PLAN: SOME SAMPLE EXERCISES

Sit, Stretch, and Strengthen

Now that you've seen how easy it is to add a little activity into your daily routine—activity that counts—you might be ready for something a little more structured. The following is an activity routine that can help you gain total body strength and flexibility. The stretching and strengthening activities are designed so that you can do them in your office or home, even while you watch TV, enjoy music, or listen to the radio. The routine is broken into three segments and takes about 30 minutes to complete. But, if you are short on time or are just beginning to do physical activity, you can do just one or two of the segments.

The routine works three separate areas of the body: the upper body, which includes shoulders, chest, and arms; the torso, which takes in the abdominal and back muscles; and the lower body, which includes the hips, legs, ankles, and feet.

If you are new to physical activity, you may want to start off by just doing one or two of these segments, especially if the full routine is more than you are able to do at first. For example, on Monday, you might do the upper body stretch and strengthen segment; on Tuesday, the torso segment; and on Wednesday, the lower body segment. Then repeat the individual segments on the following days. Another option is to do the *15-Minute Busy Day Routine* (page 131). This routine works out those muscles and joints that are typically underused as we go about our daily tasks. These joints are often prone to weakness and tightness.

Your exercise "equipment"

To get started, all you really need is a strong, stable chair, preferably without arms. Once you can comfortably do the strengthening exercises, you have the option of adding resistance in the form of an elastic band or light weights. These are items that you can purchase in most sports and fitness stores or online. They will help challenge your muscles and help you continue to build strength. Once you choose your "equipment," you'll need to keep some things in mind.

A sturdy chair

The chair should firmly support your back and the seat should be wide enough and deep enough so you are well supported and can sit comfortably. Your feet should rest fully on the floor and you should be able to position your knees comfortably over the front edge of the seat. The back of the chair should be tall enough that you can stand and hold onto it without bending or hunching over.

An exercise band (optional)

The exercise band should be long enough so that you can work against it for resistance but still do the exercises with good posture and form.

Weights (optional)

Small handheld weights, such as dumbbells, will also add resistance to your workout. But canned goods or water bottles from your pantry can serve the same purpose. Just be sure you can hold the cans or bottles comfortably in your hands. To add resistance during leg exercises, purchase weights that strap on to your ankles (see the discussion on weights below).

Adding weights to your workout

When you first begin doing strengthening activities, simply lifting your limbs in the air will probably be enough of a workout. As you become stronger, you may want to invest in some light weights. This way, you can gradually increase the amount of work you do and continue to strengthen your muscles.

Handheld weights

Dumbbells are short bars with weights fastened to each end. They typically weigh anywhere from 1 pound to 20 pounds. To start, invest in just one or two sets of dumbbells. As you gain strength, you might want to buy heavier weights as needed. Another option is to buy a set of adjustable dumbbells. Extra pounds can be added to or subtracted from these weights, allowing you to add weight as you gain strength or adjust the weight you need to use for a particular exercise. They are fairly inexpensive and don't require much storage space. Dumbbells that are covered with Neoprene are a nice option: the covering makes the weight comfortable to hold and easy to grip.

An inexpensive and easy alternative to dumbbells is to use canned goods or bottled water in a plastic container. The latter option is nice because it allows you to add or subtract weight by varying the amount of water in the container. Be certain that you can firmly hold onto any can, bottle, or other container that you use as a weight alternative; it should not be awkward to handle.

Although you may see people carrying hand weights while they are walking or jogging, this is not recommended. Carrying weights can interfere with the way your body should move and can actually cause injury.

Ankle weights

Ankle weights are padded or cushioned cuffs that wrap around your ankles and fasten securely with a strap. The cuff should not cause any rubbing or pressure points and ideally should be constructed of a smooth fabric that breathes.

The weights typically weigh anywhere from 2 to 10 pounds. The most flexible option is to purchase a set of ankle weights with pouches or straps that hold weight bars. Weight bars can then be added or subtracted to increase or decrease weight as needed.

Ankle weights are meant to provide resistance during strengthening exercises. Never use them when you are going out for a walk; they can cause joint injuries.

Caution!

Avoid using ankle weights when walking or engaging in other aerobic exercises that require a lot of leg movement. The weights can actually interfere with your normal body movements and lead to injury. Reserve ankle weights for strengthening exercises only.

Increasing the amount of weight you lift

If you have been making progress and gaining strength, you will find that you can lift more weight. Muscles become stronger by lifting heavier loads. When you are able to do 12–15 lifts easily and comfortably, you are ready to increase the amount of weight you lift. Start by adding just 1 pound.

Since you will now be lifting a heavier amount of weight, you will probably need to cut back the number of lifts you do. For example, if you have been doing 12 lifts easily, you may have to cut back to six or eight lifts when you add a 1-pound weight. Gradually work back up to doing 12–15 lifts before you add weight again.

Sit, Stretch, and Strengthen Routine

The routine below consists of a warm-up, three exercise segments, and a cool-down. You can do any one segment, two, or all three at an exercise session, but be sure to include the warm-up and cool-down whenever you exercise.

When performing the stretching and strengthening exercises that follow, keep a few tips in mind:

- ▶ Do the exercises slowly and with controlled movements. Pay attention to your body position during each exercise.
- ▶ Remember to breathe during the exercises. A general rule of thumb when lifting is to exhale on the exertion and inhale on the release. For example, during a side lateral raise, you would exhale as you bring your arms out to the side and inhale as you lower them. During a stretch, focus on breathing deeply and slowly.
- ▶ Think about the muscle you are working as you do the stretching or strengthening exercise and perform the exercise in a controlled, yet vigorous and active way.

Warm-up

Before you begin the strengthening and stretching routine, do at least a 5-minute warm-up. A good warm-up increases blood flow to your muscles and joints before you begin any activity. This will allow you to complete the routine comfortably, will reduce your risk of "pulling a muscle," and will maximize the benefit you gain from the strengthening and stretching activities. Here are ideas for ways you can warm up at home:

- ▶ march in place while you watch TV
- ▶ take a short walk around your house
- ▶ go up and down your stairs at a moderate pace
- ▶ turn on some music and dance

Stretch and Strengthen

Upper body: shoulders, chest, and arms

1. Neck and shoulder stretch

Sit up straight with your back supported by the chair and your arms down at your sides. Gently tilt your head forward toward your chest and hold for 5 seconds. Slowly roll your head to the right, bringing your right ear toward your right shoulder; hold for 5 seconds. Then roll your head forward and to the left, bringing your left ear toward your left shoulder; hold for 5 seconds. Repeat 3–5 times.

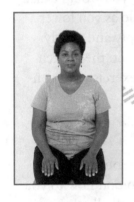
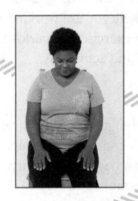
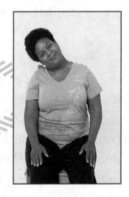
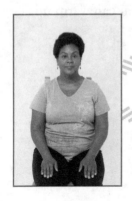
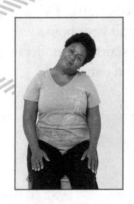

2. Shoulder shrugs

With your arms down at your sides, raise your shoulders toward your ears and slowly roll them forward and down. Repeat 5–8 times. Raise your shoulders toward your ears and slowly roll them backward and down. Repeat 5–8 times.

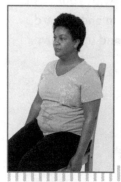 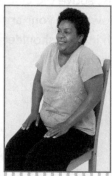 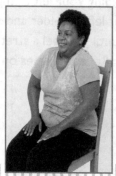 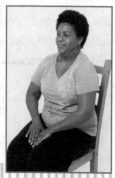

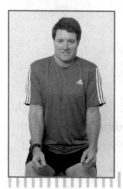 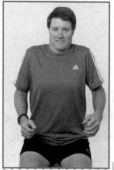 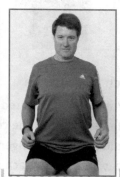 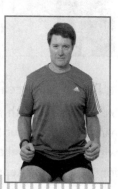

3. Shoulder, arm, and neck stretch

Hold your right arm just above the elbow with your left hand. As you look over your right shoulder, slowly pull your arm in and toward your left shoulder until you feel a stretch in your shoulder and upper arm. Hold the stretch for 10 seconds.

Switch sides, holding your left arm just above the elbow with your right hand. Look over your left shoulder and slowly pull your arm in and toward your right shoulder until you feel a stretch in your shoulder and upper arm. Hold for 10 seconds. Repeat 3 times on each side.

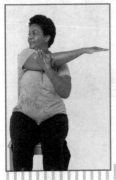 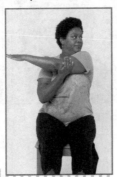

4. Reach high, reach low stretch

Sit up straight with your back supported by the chair. Reach up with your right hand, pointing your fingers toward the ceiling. At the same time, reach down with your left hand and point your fingers toward the floor. Stretch and hold for 10 seconds. Repeat 5 times for each side, alternating arms.

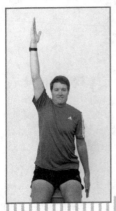 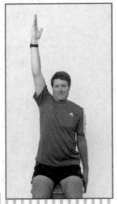

5. Triceps shoulder stretch

Reach behind your head with your left hand; place it at the top of your back between your shoulder blades. With your right hand, exert slow and gentle pressure on your left elbow until you feel a stretch in the triceps muscle, which runs under your arm from shoulder to elbow. Hold for 10 seconds. Switch sides, placing your right hand at the top of your back and exerting gentle pressure on the right elbow with your left hand. Repeat 3 times on each side, alternating arms.

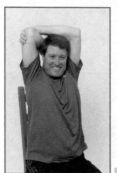 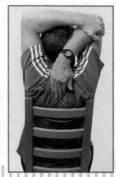 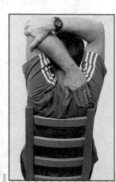

6. Arm, chest, and shoulder stretch

Sit forward in your chair with your back straight and feet firmly on the floor. Clasp your hands behind your back, just above your seat. Take a deep breath in and, keeping your elbows slightly bent, slowly "pull" your arms upward until you feel a stretch across the chest and in the arms and shoulders. Breathe naturally and think about lifting your chest upward as you stretch. Hold the stretch for 10 seconds. Repeat 3 times.

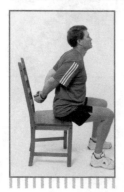

7. Biceps curl

Sit up straight with your back supported by the chair. Grasp a weight in each hand and lower your arms to your sides with your palms facing in. With your upper arms and elbows held in close to your sides, bend your elbow to curl the weight in your left hand up to thigh level. Rotate your hand to a palm-up position and continue to slowly bend your elbow until the weight reaches shoulder level. Slowly lower the weight, palm up, to thigh level. Rotate your palm so that it faces your thigh, straighten your elbow, and return the weight to the starting position. Repeat the lift 8–12 times (or as many repetitions as you find comfortable), then switch arms.

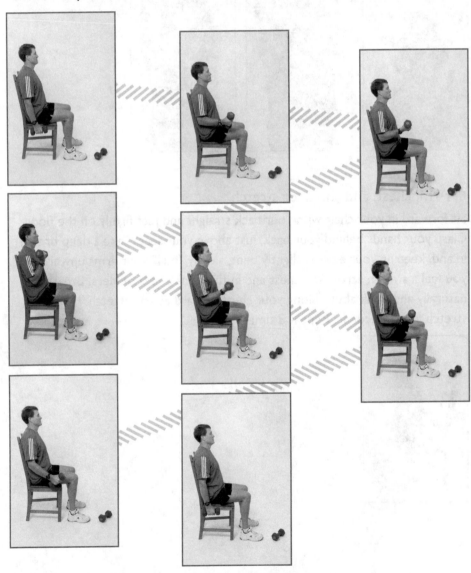

8. Triceps extension

Sit up straight with your back supported by the chair; look straight ahead and keep your chin parallel to the floor. Holding a weight in your left hand, raise it above your head; keep your arm straight, with the elbow facing forward and your upper arm close to your ear. With your right hand, grasp the back of your left upper arm just below the elbow for support. Slowly bend your elbow and lower the weight toward your left shoulder. Return to the starting position. Do 8–12 repetitions with your left arm, then switch arms.

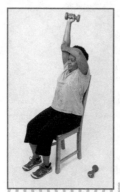 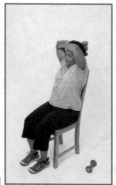 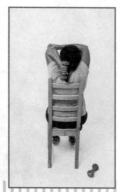

Key points to remember!

▶ For all lifting activities use slow, controlled movements (count slowly 1, 2, 3, 4, 5 as you lift, and then repeat the count as you bring the weight down).
▶ Exhale as you lift the weight and inhale as you return your arm to the starting position.

9. Side lateral raise

Sit forward in your chair with your feet firmly on the floor. Grasp a weight in each hand and lower your arms to your sides with your palms facing in. Keeping your elbows slightly bent, slowly raise both arms out to the side until your hands are just above shoulder level. (This is your goal; if you cannot reach to shoulder level, simply lift to a comfortable position for you.) Pause, then slowly lower your arms to the starting position. Remember to exhale as you lift the weight and inhale as you lower it. Repeat 8–12 times.

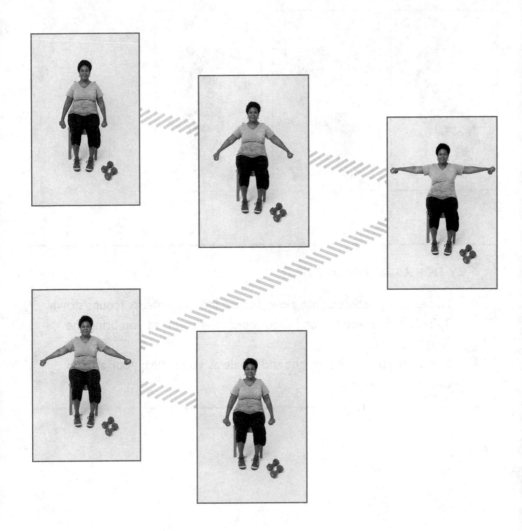

▶ If raising both arms at the same time is too difficult, try this method: Keeping your body straight in the chair, hold onto the side of your chair with one hand. With a weight in the other hand, do 8–12 lifts, then switch and do the exercise with the opposite arm.

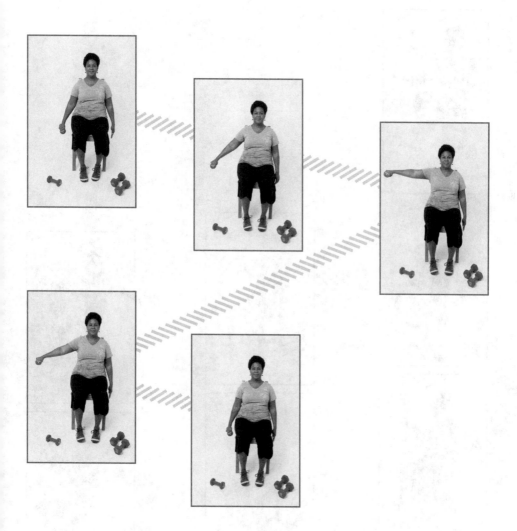

10. Seated chest fly (performed with exercise band)

Sit up straight with your back supported by the chair. Hold one end of an exercise band in each hand and raise your arms straight up over your head. Now lower the band behind your head and position it across your back, just below your shoulder blades. Keeping your elbows slightly bent, straighten your arms out to either side. Then slowly bring your arms forward until your forearms meet in front of your chest. Exhale as you bring the arms in, and inhale as you slowly return your arms out to the side. Repeat 8–12 times.

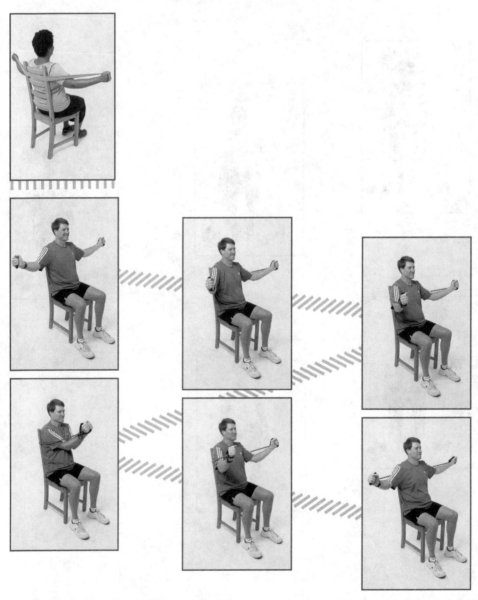

Torso: abdominals and back

11. Side stretch

Sit up straight in your chair, with the hips slightly forward from the chair back and feet placed firmly on the floor. Keeping your hips in a forward position, turn your upper body to the right. As you look over your right shoulder, grasp the chair back and gently pull against it until you feel a stretch in your left side. Hold the stretch for 10–15 seconds. Repeat the stretch 2–3 times, alternating sides.

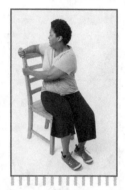

12. Abdominal brace

Sit forward in your chair with your feet placed firmly on the floor. Place one hand on either side of the seat of your chair next to your hips. Pull your shoulders upward, straightening your posture. Take a breath in and relax your stomach muscles. Breathe out and draw your lower stomach muscles inward (visualize that you are pulling your navel back toward your spine). Hold this position for 5–10 seconds. Focus on relaxed breathing; avoid holding your breath while your muscles are contracting. Repeat 5 times.

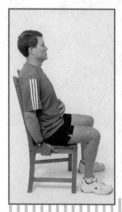
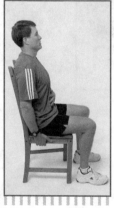

13. Chair sit-up

Sit up straight in your chair with your feet firmly on the floor, arms bent at your sides, and hands in front of your chest with palms facing forward (as if you are going to push something). Slowly bend forward at the waist, pulling in your abdominal muscles and keeping your back straight. As you bend forward, extend your elbows and push out with your hands, exhaling as you go. Slowly come up and return to the starting position. Repeat 8–12 times.

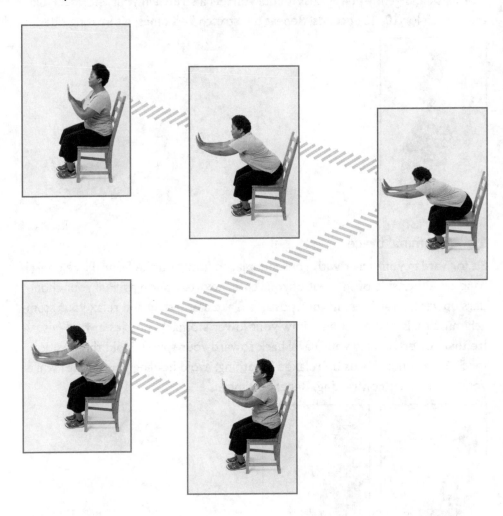

14. Seated abdominal curl

Sit forward in your chair with your hips toward the front edge of the seat. Lean back so that your upper back is supported by the back of the chair. Hold onto the sides of the seat for support and extend your legs out in front of you. Keep your knees slightly bent, heels on the floor, and toes up. Cross your left ankle over your right, pull in your abdominal muscles, and slowly lift your feet 2–3 inches off the floor (the effort to lift should come from your abdominal muscles, not your hips). Pause, and then slowly lower your legs to the starting position. Repeat for 8–12 lifts, then cross your right ankle over your left and repeat.

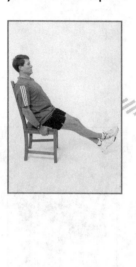
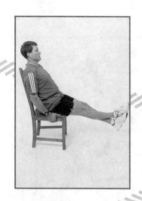
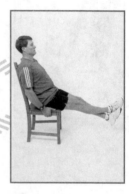
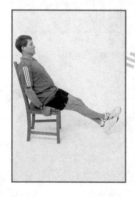

15. Seated lower back/cat stretch

Sit up straight in your chair, feet firmly on the floor. Slowly bend forward, lowering your chest toward your thighs; let your arms dangle toward your feet. Hold the stretch for 10–15 seconds, then round your upper back, tuck your chin toward your chest, and lift your upper body halfway to the starting position; continue to let your arms dangle toward your feet. Hold this position for 10–15 seconds, then put your hands on your thighs and slowly lift your upper body to the starting position. Repeat 3 times.

> ▶ If you have retinopathy or have been advised to limit head-low activities and posture changes for any other health reason, check with your physician before you do this stretch.

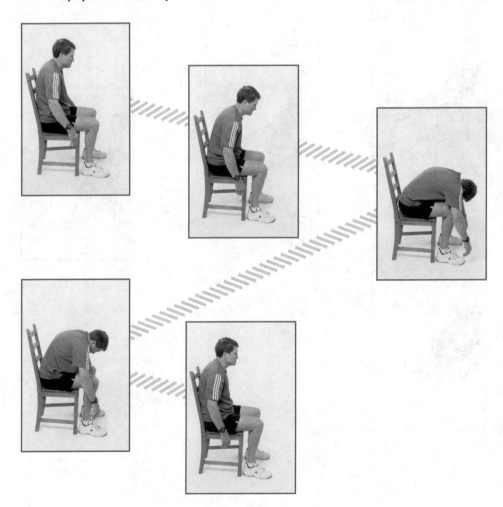

16. Reverse chair sit-up

Sit up straight in your chair, hips at the back of the seat, feet firmly on the floor, and hands lightly gripping the sides of the chair for support. While keeping your back straight, bend forward, chest toward thighs. Slowly straighten up to a seated position with your back supported by the chair. Repeat 8–12 times.

▶ To increase the resistance, loop an exercise band under the arches of your feet (always wear shoes), and hold one end of the band in each hand. Bend your elbows and anchor your hands against your chest, palms in. Bend forward and then slowly straighten to a seated position with your back supported by the chair. Repeat 8–12 times.

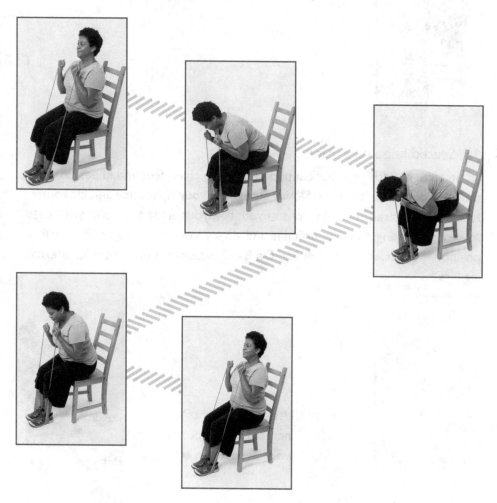

17. Knee to chest stretch

Sit up straight with your back supported by the chair, feet on the floor. Clasp your hands around your left knee and slowly pull your knee up toward your chest; hold for 10–15 seconds. Repeat 3 times. Repeat sequence with your right leg.

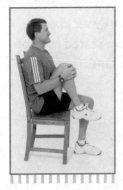

18. Seated knee extension

Sit up straight with your back supported by the chair, feet and knees positioned shoulder-width apart. Slowly straighten your right knee and lift your foot until it is straight out in front of you; flex your ankle and point your toes toward the ceiling. Relax your ankle and slowly lower your leg to the starting position. Repeat with your left leg. Do 8–12 extensions on each side, alternating legs.

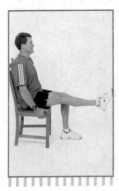

▶ Use ankle weights to increase the amount of work as you gain strength.

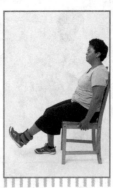

19. Seated hamstring stretch

Sit up straight with your back supported by the chair. Keep your right foot on the floor while you extend your left leg out in front of you with the heel on the floor, toes pointing up. Keeping your back straight, slowly bend forward, bringing your upper body toward your left knee. Gently hold your lower left leg with your hands. Hold the stretch for 10–15 seconds. Repeat the stretch 3 times on the left leg, and then switch legs.

▶ If you have been advised to avoid posture changes or "head-low" activities, you may use a foot stool, ottoman, or another chair when you do this stretch. Extend your leg and place the lower leg and heel on the stool or ottoman, toes pointed up. Be certain your leg is well supported.

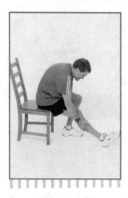

20. Standing hip extension

Stand about 1 1/2 feet behind your chair and hold onto the back for support. Bend forward at the waist with a slight angle. Look straight ahead, keeping your head, neck, and torso in a straight line. Bend your right knee slightly for support, then slowly lift your left leg behind you until your leg and torso are aligned; your toes should be 8–12 inches from the floor and pointed down toward it. Slowly return your leg to the starting position. Repeat with your right leg. Do 8–12 lifts on each side, alternating legs.

▶ You may add ankle weights to increase the amount of work as you gain strength.

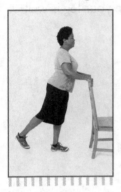

21. Standing side hip raise

Stand 4–6 inches behind your chair and hold on to the back for support. Keeping your toes pointed forward and your leg straight, slowly lift your right leg out to the side until it is about 6 inches off the floor. Keep the knee of the supporting leg slightly bent and your torso upright. Pause at the top of the lift, then return your right leg to its starting position. Do 8–12 lifts on each side, alternating legs.

▶ You may use ankle weights to increase the amount of work as you gain strength.

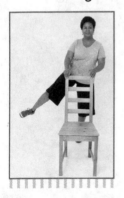

22. Seated foot and toe stretches

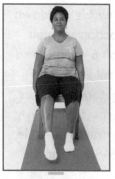

A. Sit up straight with your back supported by the chair and your feet on the floor. Lift one heel off the floor, point your toes, and extend them forward and downward until you feel a mild stretch; hold for 10–15 seconds. Return to starting position and repeat with the other foot.

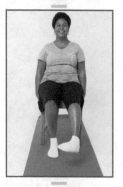

B. Rest one heel on the floor, then slowly flex your ankle and pull your toes up so they point toward the ceiling; hold for 10–15 seconds. Return to starting position and repeat with the other foot.

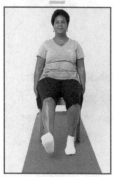

C. With your feet flat on the floor, lift the toes of one foot 1–2 inches off the floor. Rotate your toes in so they point toward your opposite foot; hold for 10–15 seconds. Return to starting position and repeat with the other foot.

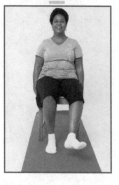

D. With your feet flat on the floor, lift the toes of one foot 1–2 inches off the floor. Rotate your toes out and away from your other foot; hold for 10–15 seconds. Return to starting position and repeat with the other foot.

23. Ankle circles

Lift your left foot about two inches off the floor and point your big toe down toward the floor. Next, rotate your ankle in a clockwise direction as if you are drawing a circle with your toe. Repeat this circular motion 6–8 times in a clockwise direction. Next switch directions and rotate your ankle in a counterclockwise circle 6–8 times. Now, switch feet. Lift your right foot 2 inches off the floor, point your big toe down toward the floor, and rotate your right ankle 6–8 times in a counterclockwise direction as if you are drawing a circle with your toe. Then switch directions and circle your ankle 6–8 times in a clockwise direction.

24. Toe stand

Stand 12 inches behind the back of your chair with your feet shoulder width apart; hold onto the back of the chair for support. Slowly raise your heels off the floor and lift up onto the balls of your feet. Pause, and then slowly lower your heels to the starting position. Repeat 8–12 times.

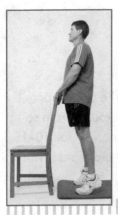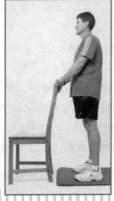

25. Heel stand

For this last exercise, use a wall for support. Stand with your back against the wall, arms down at your sides, and the palms of your hands against the wall. Place your heels a few inches out from the wall, then slowly raise your toes off the floor and balance on your heels. Pause, and then slowly lower your toes to the starting position. Repeat 8–12 times.

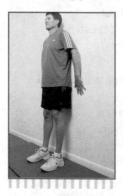

Cool-down

Just as you began this routine with a warm-up, it is important to end it with a good 5-minute cool-down. The purpose of a cool-down period is to allow your body to gradually get used to a resting state after activity. To cool down, simply repeat a few of the stretches from the sit and stretch routine. This will help minimize any muscle soreness or tightness after you are done. At the end of the cool-down, it is nice to sit back in your chair, close your eyes, take some deep breaths in and out, and focus on how good you feel!

Sit, Stretch, and Strengthen Summary Sheet

Warm-up (5 minutes)
Stretch and Strengthen

Upper body: shoulders, chest, and arms
1. Neck and shoulder stretch
2. Shoulder shrugs
3. Shoulder, arm, and neck stretch
4. Reach high, reach low stretch
5. Triceps shoulder stretch
6. Arm, chest, and shoulder stretch
7. Biceps curl
8. Triceps extension
9. Side lateral raise
10. Seated chest fly

Torso: abdominals and back
11. Side stretch
12. Abdominal brace
13. Chair sit-up
14. Seated abdominal curl
15. Seated lower back/cat stretch
16. Reverse chair sit-up

Lower body: hips, legs, ankles, and feet
17. Knee to chest stretch
18. Seated knee extension
19. Seated hamstring stretch
20. Standing hip extension
21. Standing side hip raise
22. Seated foot and toe stretches
23. Ankle circles
24. Toe stand
25. Heel stand

Cool-down (5 minutes)

Tips to remember:
When you stretch:
▶ Hold the stretch for 10–30 seconds
▶ Focus on relaxed breathing, avoid breath holding
▶ Keep it comfortable
▶ Avoid bouncing or bobbing

When you strengthen:
▶ Do slow, controlled movements (count 1,2,3,4,5 up/out then 1,2,3,4,5 down/in)
▶ Focus on breathing (breathe out as you push or lift; breathe in as you return to the relaxed, starting position)
▶ Keep it comfortable
▶ Start slowly and gradually build up. (The suggested number of repetitions of an exercise are goals. If you are not able to do this many at first, start with fewer (4–6) repetitions and gradually increase the number that you do. When you feel mild muscle discomfort, this is a good indication that you have done enough.)
▶ Always ask your physician if you are uncertain whether a stretch or strengthening activity is a safe activity for you

15-Minute Busy Day Routine

Warm-up (5 minutes)
Stretch and Strengthen

Upper body: shoulders, chest, and arms
1. Neck and shoulder stretch
2. Shoulder shrugs
3. Shoulder, arm, and neck stretch
5. Triceps shoulder stretch
8. Triceps extension
9. Side lateral raise

Torso: abdominals and back
11. Side stretch
12. Abdominal brace
15. Seated lower back/cat stretch
16. Reverse chair sit-up

Lower body: hips, legs, ankles, and feet
17. Knee to chest stretch
19. Seated hamstring stretch
20. Standing hip extension
21. Standing side hip raise
22. Seated foot and toe stretches

Cool-down (5 minutes)

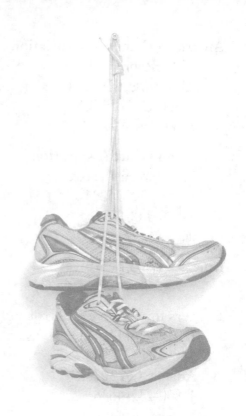

APPENDIX 1

Physical Activity, Diabetes and Health Resources

Organizations, Associations, and Agencies

Academy of Nutrition and Dietetics
120 South Riverside Plaza, Suite 2000
Chicago, IL 60606-6995
www.eatright.org

American College of Sports Medicine
402 West Michigan St.
Indianapolis, IN 46202-9200
1-317-637-9200
www.acsm.org

American Diabetes Association
1701 Beauregard St.
Alexandria, VA 22311
1-800-DIABETES
www.diabetes.org

American Heart Association
7272 Greenville Ave.
Dallas, TX 75231
1-800-242-8721
www.heart.org

America On The Move
www.americaonthemove.org

Centers for Disease Control and Prevention
Division of Diabetes Translation
1600 Clifton Rd.
Atlanta, GA 30333
1-800-232-4636
www.cdc.gov/diabetes

Division of Nutrition, Physical Activity and Obesity
1600 Clifton Rd.
Atlanta, GA 30333
1-800-232-4636
www.cdc.gov/nccdphp/dnpa

Insulin dependence
249 S. Hwy 101, #8000
San Diego, CA 92075-1807
1-888-912-3837
www.insulindependence.org

National Diabetes Prevention Program
1600 Clifton Rd.
Atlanta, GA 30333
1-800-232-6348
www.cdc.gov/diabetes/prevention/

National Diabetes Education Program
One Diabetes Way
Bethesda, MD 20814-9692
1-800-438-5383
www.ndep.nih.gov

National Diabetes Information Clearinghouse
NIDDK, NIH
Bldg. 31, Rm. 9A06
31 Center Dr., MSC 2560
Bethesda, MD 20893-2560
1-301-496-3583
http://www.diabetes.niddk.nih.gov

Go4Life: National Institute on Aging at NIH
NIOA
Bldg. 31, Rm. 5C27
31 Center Dr., MSC 2292
Bethesda, MD 20892
1-800-222-2225
http://go4life.niapublications.org/

Physical Activity Guidelines for Americans:
National Health Information Center
P.O. Box 1133
Washington, DC 20013-1133
1-800-336-4794
http://www.health.gov/paguidelines/

Shape Up America!
www.shapeup.org

Publications

ACSM Fitness Book
American College of Sports Medicine
Human Kinetics
P.O. Box 5076
Champaign, IL 61825-5076
1-800-747-4457
http://www.Humankinetics.com

Exercise: *A Guide from the National Institute on Aging*
NIH Publication No. 01-4258
1-800-222-2225
http://www.nia.nih.gov/publication/exer

Small Steps. Big Rewards. *Your GAME PLAN to Prevent Type 2 Diabetes*
National Diabetes Education Program
One Diabetes Way
Bethesda, MD 20814-9692
1-888-963-6337
http://www.ndep.nih.gov/publications/PubId=71

The Step Diet Book
James O. Hill PhD, John C. Peters PhD,
    Bonnie T. Jortberg MS, RD & Pamela Peeke, MD
Workman Publishing (2004)

The 7 Step Diabetes Fitness Plan
Sheri R. Colberg PhD
Marlow & Company (2006)
http://shericolberg.com/diabetes-fitness

DVDs

Armchair Fitness
7755 16th St. NW
Washington, DC 20012
1-800-453-6280
www.armchairfitness.com/info.html

Go4Life Everyday Exercise from the National Institute on Aging
NIOA
Bldg. 31, Rm. 5C27
31 Center Dr., MSC 2292
Bethesda, MD 20892
1-800-222-4225
http://go4life.niapublications.org/exercise-guide-video

LifeSpan Fitness Forever
Informative and balanced fitness routine based on sound exercise principles. Follows the American College of Sports Medicine Position Stand Recommendations "Exercise and Physical Activity for Older Adults."
LifeSpan Fitness
Fitness Forever
P.O. Box 981316
Park City, UT 84098-1316
1-877-654-EVER
www.fitnessforever.com

Walk Aerobics videos with Leslie Sansone
Walk aerobics DVDs offer options for everyone from beginning exercisers to those who have a good fitness foundation and are able to walk at a moderate-brisk pace for 30 minutes or more. More advanced routines include movements that require good balance and agility. A 40 Plus Workout Walk Aerobics and a Senior Aerobics DVD (www.lesliesansonvideos.com/senioraerobics.htm) are also available. Be sure to check out "Walk Down Your Blood Sugar," too. It is an excellent resource for people with diabetes.
Fitness Gurus
848 N. Rainbow Blvd. #4164
Las Vegas, NV 89107
www.lesliesansonevideos.com

Websites

Diabetes Healthsense: Resources for Healthy Living
This site, brought to you by the National Diabetes Education Program, provides easy access to resources to help you live well and meet your fitness and health goals—whether you have diabetes, pre-diabetes, or risk factors for the disease.
http://www.ndep.nih.gov/resources/diabetes-healthsense/?redirect=true

Physical Activity Guidelines for Americans
This website contains a wealth of information and offers sound guidance on the types and amounts of physical activity that provide substantial health benefits for Americans. The main idea behind the Guidelines is that regular physical activity over months and years can produce long-term health benefits.
http://www.health.gov/paguidelines/

Tips for Evaluating Websites

Questions to ask when evaluating health and fitness information on the internet:

- ▶ What type of website is it?
  - ▶ .com or commercial site (often selling a product or service)
  - ▶ .edu or educational (university or college) site
  - ▶ .gov or government agency site
  - ▶ .org or organization (nonprofit, not for profit, or for profit) site
- ▶ Who are the authors?
  - ▶ Are they listed?
  - ▶ What are their credentials, including professional certifications and/or licenses?
  - ▶ What is their occupation or employment experience?
  - ▶ Will they gain financially from the information included on the website? Note: Authors of .com sites are often trying to sell something and may be financially motivated.

▶ What is the purpose of the website?
  ▷ to inform or explain?
  ▷ to present an opinion or promote a cause?
  ▷ to persuade?
  ▷ to sell?
▶ How reliable is the information included on the site?
  ▷ Is an original source or reference for the information given?
  ▷ What is the original source of the information—book, professional journal, magazine, or newspaper?
  ▷ What institution supports or represents the information—academic institution, government agency, health organization, or private company? Or is this a personal Web page?
  ▷ How current is the information and when was the site last updated?

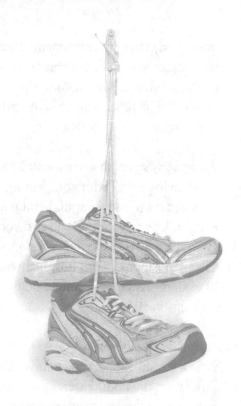

APPENDIX 2

Simple Physical Fitness Self-Assessment

Here is a basic self-assessment routine that you can do to check your own physical fitness. As you can see, there aren't any strict guidelines. This is simply a way for you to check your progress as you move forward with your activity routine. Repeat this self-assessment every month and keep track of improvements in your level of fitness (check with your physician to make sure all of these assessment activities are safe for you to do).

Start each assessment with 5 minutes of easy warm-up walking and some light stretching.

Cardiorespiratory endurance assessment: 5-minute timed walk
Walk for 5 minutes and see how far you can go (maintain a moderate level of effort). You can measure step counts, laps around your house or yard, or distance up and down your street. As you become fitter, you should be able to walk farther in the same 5-minute time interval.

Lower body strength assessment: 30-second chair stand

Sit in a sturdy, supportive chair with your feet flat on the floor, about 1 foot apart, and your hands on your hips. Count how many times you can come to a full stand in 30 seconds. As you gain strength, you should be able to stand more times in 30 seconds.

Upper body strength assessment: 30-second wall push-up

Stand facing a wall with your feet together, with your arms extended and hands pressed flat against the wall. Bend your elbows and, while keeping your back straight, lean toward the wall as if you are going to touch it with your nose. Then straighten your elbows and push your body away from the wall to your starting position. Count how many times you can repeat this wall push-up in 30 seconds. As you gain upper body strength, you should be able to do more push-ups in 30 seconds.

Flexibility: Sit and reach

Sit in a sturdy, supportive chair with its back braced against a wall. Place one foot flat on the floor. Extend your other leg outward and place the heel of your foot on the floor with your toes pointing upward. Reach with your hands toward the toes of your extended leg. Notice how far you are able to reach your fingertips either short of or beyond your toes. Then switch legs and repeat the assessment. As you become more flexible, you should be able to reach farther.

Balance assessment: One-leg stand

(Note: Stand near a countertop to steady yourself in case you lose your balance.) Stand on one foot, without support for as long as possible. Switch legs and repeat on the opposite side. Note how long you are able to stand without losing your balance. The length of time that you can stand on one foot should increase with practice.

INDEX

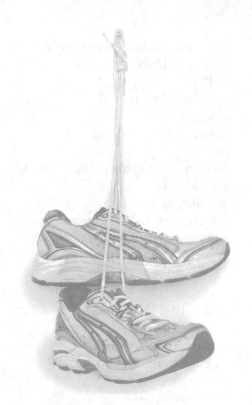

Note: Page numbers followed by an *f* refer to figures. Page numbers followed by a *t* refer to tables. Page numbers in **bold** refer to in-depth discussions.

alpha-glucosidase inhibitors, 88*t*
American Diabetes Association, 98, 134
ankle weights, 108, 124
ankles, 124–131
anxiety, 7
appetite, 7
apps (applications), 15, 98, 110–118
arm, 130–131
arthritis, 9*t*
associations, 133–135
autonomic neuropathy, 8, 9*t*

B

back, 119–123, 130–131
balance, 34, 37
balance assessment, 142
baseline minutes (walking), 99
biguanides, 88*t*
blood fat levels, 8
blood glucose
    control, 84–91
    goals, 78*f*–79*f*
    levels, 59, 66, 76–77, 84–86, 87*t*, 93. *see also* hyperglycemia; hypoglycemia
    management, 4–6, 74, **83–93**
    monitoring, 75–76
    patterns, 76
    record, 78*f*–79*f*
blood pressure, 6. *See also* high blood pressure
body composition, 61, 63, 65–69
bone fracture, 34
Borg Rating of Perceived Exertion (RPE) Scale, 28–29, 33–34
breathing, 109, 115

C

calisthenics, 34, 69–71

calories, 7, 14, 43*t*, 44–46, 67–69
car travel, 52
carbohydrate (CHO), 87, 89–90, 91*t*
cardiorespiratory endurance assessment, 141
cardiorespiratory fitness, 61, 64–65
cardiovascular health, 4, 6, 66, 83, 85
cell phone. *See* smartphone
chair, 106. *See also* sitting; *specific seated exercises*
chest, 110–118, 130–131
cholesterol levels, 6, 83
Choose My Plate, 14
circulation. *See* peripheral vascular disease
circulatory system, 61
clothing, 92, 96
combination medication, 88*t*
commitment, 21–22, 58, 103
Confidence Scale, 11–12
contract, 22, 23*f*
cooking/baking, 44
cool-down, 72, 92, 109, 129–131
coronary artery disease (CAD), 8
cost/benefit balance sheet, 25–27
cues, 27

D

Daily Diabetes Self-Management Record, 78*f*–79*f*, 81*f*
dehydration, 85
diabetes
    A1c, 74
    body weight risk, 65
    complications, 8, 9*t*
    equipment, 93
    exercise and, 5
    identification, 93
    management, 75–76, 85
    prevention, 74
    safety considerations, 93
    supplies, 53

M

management plan, 74–82
medical support team, 7, 46, 60–61, 62t–63t, 65t, 73, 84–86, 93, 101
medication, 75–76, 78f–79f, 84, 86, 88t, 93. *See also specific medication*
metabolic rate, 7
moderate activities, 43t, 45t, 46, 61, 67–68, 73t, 85, 92
muscle, 5–7, 32–36, 61, 63, 86, 109
muscle strength, 63, 69–71, 73t
muscle strengthening activities, 4, 39

N

negative thoughts, 24
nephropathy, 8, 9t
nerve damage. *See* autonomic neuropathy; peripheral neuropathy
nutrition, 13–14. *See also* eating/ eating plan

O

oral medication, 88t
organizations, 133–135
osteoporosis, 9t, 34

P

pace, 73–74, 100–102
pedometer, 97–99
peripheral neuropathy, 8, 9t
peripheral vascular disease, 8, 9t
Physical Activity Guidelines for Americans, 3, 8, 59, 138
physical fitness, 61
physical fitness self-assessment, 141–142
physically active/inactive jobs, 49t

planning, 28, 53–55, **105–131**
play, 44–48
positive thinking, 25t
posture, 102
pre-diabetes, 4–6, 65–66, 74, 86
pre-exercise health assessment, 62t–63t
premature heart disease, 8
publications, 136
pulling, 35, 39
pulse count, 69f
pushing, 35, 39

Q

quick-fix thinking, 57–58

R

record keeping, 76–77, 78f, 79–80, 82, 103
relaxation, 36–37
resistance exercise, 34–36, 39, 67, 69–71
resources, 98, 133–139
restaurant eating, 50
retinopathy, 8, 9t
reward, 19, 59, 103
RPE (rating of perceived exertion), 64, 67, 72, 73t

S

safety considerations, 92–93
self-confidence, 11
self-contract, 59
self-management, 83–84
self-monitoring, 28–29
session, 38, 59–60, 75–76
shoes, 51, 92, 96
shoulder, 110–118, 130–131
sickness, 78f–79f, 84–85